GABOR PALOS

SIMPLIFIED LINDY HOP
FOR MEN

Gabor Palos

Simplified Lindy Hop
for Men

GABOR PALOS

SIMPLIFIED LINDY HOP FOR MEN

First Edition 2024

ISBN 978-1-7770046-1-3

Table of Contents

Introduction

This book is a guide for those wanting to learn the leader's part of the dance called Lindy Hop. It includes general information on swing music and swing dancing, basic and intermediate Lindy Hop steps and figures, Charleston steps, jazz or "break" steps, footwork variations, dancing to fast and slow music and tips on learning, practicing and social dancing.

The emphasis is not on a detailed technical description of the figures included in the book. Such descriptions are often laborious and difficult to read, and further information on each step is readily available in group classes or online videos. As such, the description of the steps in this book is aimed at being simple and practical.

The main purpose of this book is to give the reader an overall sense of the process of learning the dance, to provide background information on the history and the main building blocks of the dance, suggest a list of the most useful steps to learn, tips on how to execute these steps, how to shape and lead a dance and how to practice and grow your skills.

Enjoy learning and dancing the Lindy Hop!

February 2024

Swing and the Lindy Hop

Origins of the dance

The dance called Lindy Hop was created in the mid-1920s in Harlem, New York by African-American dancers from elements taken from other dances that preceded it, primarily the Breakaway, the Charleston and tap dancing. The emerging new dance was unofficially named after Charles Lindbergh who crossed ("hopped") the Atlantic Ocean with the first ever solo, non-stop flight from New York to Paris in 1927. The main venue for the new dance was the Savoy Ballroom on Lenox Avenue in Harlem (sadly, the ballroom was demolished in 1959).

Two main styles of Lindy Hop emerged in the 1930s and 1940s: first the "Savoy-style", mainly danced by African-American dancers in Harlem, and later the "Hollywood" or "LA-style" (also called "smooth" style), mainly danced by white dancers on the West Coast, in California.

Those who want to understand the origins and history of Lindy Hop should read two autobiographical books by two of the original Savoy dancers: "*Swingin' at the Savoy, The Memoir of A Jazz Dancer*" by Norma Miller (Temple University Press, 1996) and "*Ambassador of Lindy Hop*" by Frankie Manning (Temple University Press, 2007).

For visual reference, old film footage, generally available online, offer a glimpse into how these original swing dances were danced. A good example of such old recordings is Part 1 of the three-part documentary "*The Spirit Moves*". A more show-oriented performance of Lindy Hop can be seen in the 1937 movie "*A Day at the Races*".

2

With the advent of television in the 1950s and '60s, social partner dancing gradually disappeared from mainstream entertainment and spent a few decades in hibernation. In the 1980s, Lindy Hop was re-discovered by a group of dancers in America, Britain and Sweden who studied the dance from old movie clips and engaged still living old-timers from the 1930s to teach it.

Partner dancing is still not a mainstream form of entertainment for the general public but those interested can find their local community of like-minded dancers, at least in urban centres.

Today, the closest "living relatives" of Lindy Hop are the East Coast Swing, Jive, Balboa, the St. Louis Shag and the Collegiate Shag. East Coast Swing and Jive are simplified and standardised ballroom versions of the Lindy Hop, adapted to the needs of franchised commercial dance studios. These two (nearly identical) dances are almost entirely "6-count" based and most of their steps can be incorporated into Lindy Hop. Another dance, the West Coast Swing has "swing" in its name, but it is generally not danced to swing music.

Nature of the dance

Only by knowing something about the history of the dance will become clear why Lindy Hop instruction, somewhat confusingly, consists of variously teaching "Lindy steps", "Charleston steps" and "solo jazz (or 'break') steps". In social dancing these three types of steps are mixed to add variety and fun to the dance. Many figures can be danced with "normal footwork" or alternatively with "Charleston footwork" (which involves a lot of "kicking"), or embellished with footwork borrowed from jazz and tap dancing.

If this is not confusing enough, even the basic rhythm pattern of the Lindy Hop is not constant. Most figures are "8-count" and follow a 1-2-3&4-5-6-7&8 pattern, but plenty of figures are "6-count" and follow a 1-2-3&4-5&6 pattern. Many steps have both 6- and 8-

count versions. Jazz steps and "repetitive" type of steps can last any (even) number of beats.

There are no rules to say when 6- or 8-count figures should be danced. Any of them can be danced at any time. Generally speaking, if you are looking for rules in Lindy Hop, you are out of luck. You will know that you are becoming an experienced dancer when you no longer need to count your steps and you are still able to fit your dance to the music. Ultimately it is the music that drives the dance, and the two basic rhythm patterns, as well as jazz steps and repetitive steps can be freely mixed during dancing as long as they respond to the rhythm of the music. Developing a sense of what the music calls for takes time and experience.

Mixing Lindy, Charleston and break steps while constantly switching between 8-, 6-, and other count patterns make Lindy Hop a challenging dance, but it also prevents Lindy Hop from ever becoming boring.

Swing music

Lindy Hop is a swing dance, which means that it is meant to be danced to swing music. It is still danced mostly to the swing music of the 1920s and '30s or to contemporary swing music emulating that era. To understand Lindy Hop, one should have a basic understanding of swing music.

Swing was the most popular type of jazz music in the United States from the 1930s to the mid-1940s. It was played by large bands consisting of up to fifty musicians. It was mostly written music, in contrast to the improvised nature of other jazz styles.

"Swing music" has never been clearly defined and it is somewhat difficult to explain, although you will generally recognize it when you hear it. A characteristic feature of swing music is the emphasis

4

on the off-beat or weaker pulse in the music in relation to fixed beats, and a particular "swing-time" or "swung" rhythm pattern.

"Swung rhythm" can be best understood in comparison to "straight rhythm". In straight rhythm (or timing) an off-beat note is placed evenly between two fixed beats, but in swing rhythm it is placed closer to the second beat. For example both Cha Cha and Lindy Hop have a basic "step-step-triple-step" (1-2-3&4) pattern, but in Cha Cha the "&" is evenly placed between 3 and 4, while in Lindy Hop it is closer to 4.

Although Lindy Hop triple-steps are generally danced in swung rhythm, occasionally straight rhythm can be used for "runs", either to cover more space, or to add variety by breaking the typical pattern of the dance.

As a footwork variation, the typical swung rhythm of the Lindy Hop triple step can be changed so that the middle step is closer (in time) to the first than to the third step, i.e. "3-&4" becomes "3&-4".

The timing and structure of a song

Swing music is generally written in 4/4 ("four-four") time which is the most common meter of timing in music, and for this reason it is also called "common time". 4/4 means that there are four one-quarter note beats (4/4 = 4 x ¼) in each measure (or "bar") of music. In other words, when a song in 4/4 time is put to paper, it is broken down into small groups of 4 one-quarter note beats. The composer may also use half notes, eighth notes etc but all of these together must add up to 4/4 in each bar of music. The bar is the most important basic building block of a piece of music or song.

In response to the time constraints of studio recording, commercial swing music has developed a few relatively simple compositional structures. Each piece of swing music has a certain typical (although flexible) structure or composition, just like various forms of poetry have their typical structures. Knowing this, a dancer may choose his steps and dancing so as to better mirror or respond to the structure of the music.

The musical units, or building blocks of a piece of swing music are the "beat", the "bar", the "phrase" and the "chorus". As just mentioned, each bar of music contains four (quarter note) beats. Eight bars (32 beats) of music typically form a musical "phrase" (which can be thought of as a line in a poem), and four phrases typically form a "chorus" (which can be thought of as a verse). This structure is flexible. In addition, the song may start with a short introduction.

Even though the basic unit of a song is one bar (4 beats), a typical melody is written over 2 bars (8 beats), largely because 4 beats are too short to create a melody. Because of this, a dancer will usually perceive a musical phrase as four sets of 8-count sections (rather than eight 4-count bars).

Each phrase generally follows a certain pattern where, for example, the same melody is repeated three times, followed by a different melody in the fourth 8-count section. The pattern of such a phrase would be AAAB. Other patterns may also be used.

A dancer could then choose, for example, to dance an "AAAB" phrase with Swingouts on the A's and a Freeze or a Lindy Circle on the B, or choose some other way to mark the distinction between the A and B sections.

Similarly to the phrases, each chorus of the music also generally follows a certain pattern where, for example, the same melody is repeated twice over two phrases, followed by a different melody in the third phrase, then returning to the original melody in the fourth phrase. The pattern of such a chorus would be AABA.

A dancer could then, for example, choose to dance to an "AABA" type chorus with Lindy Hop figures on the A's and Charleston steps on the B.

Finally, the choruses that make up the song also usually follow a pattern that can be AABA, or something else. The dancer may find a way to respond to this distinction as well.

Any such pattern or regularity in the song structure can be used to drive the choice of dance moves. With time, one will develop an ear to spot the structure of a song and the ability to design his dance around that pattern. Being in sync with the music does not only look good, if feels good as well.

Counting the beats

When the Lindy Hop was born back in the 1930s, dancers were not counting the beats in a figure. Purists still frown at applying "counting" to the figures and believe that one should learn to dance "naturally", just as one learns their mother tongue. But whether one acknowledges it or not, music does have a structure, figures do have a count, and it does not hurt to try to understand what goes on when you are dancing.

The figures in Lindy Hop typically cover either 8 beats of music ("8-count steps") or 6 beats of music ("6-count steps"). Other, repetitive type of figures may cover any (even) number of beats. This variety of counts makes it a challenge to match the dance to the music because it can change the timing of the moves relative to the phrasing of the music, resulting in a mismatch.

An 8-count figure covers two bars of music, so if you danced only 8-count figures, you would always be in sync with the music. 6-count figures have a bit of a problem in that they occupy only 1.5 bars, so you have to pay attention to combining 6 and 8-count moves in a certain way if you want the end of a figure to coincide with the end of a musical phrase.

If we break down the rhythm and the figures even further, we find that "2 beats" is the ultimate basic unit of the dance. Any particular figure is a set of 2-beat moves, and for that reason any figure can be interrupted and changed into something else at ever second beat.

Although pne should not be obsessed with counting the beats, you should still strive to dance "to the music", because when your dancing is in harmony with the music, this harmony is felt both by you, your dance partner, and those watching you dance.

"Straight steps" and "change steps"

If you look at it this way, there are only two kinds of dance figures: one ends with your weight on the same foot where you started from (I will call these "straight steps") and the other ends with your weight on the other foot (I will call these "change steps"). A straight figure contains an even number of weight changes (or no weight change). A change figure contains an odd number of weight changes.

For example the rock step, the Kick-Ball-Change, kick-and-hold, and the simple "hold" are straight steps. The single step, triple step and kick-step are examples of change steps.

It is useful to be aware which steps are straight or change, so that you can vary your dance and still end up on the "correct" foot that allows you to proceed to your next step or figure.

Straight steps are interchangeable among themselves, and change steps are interchangeable among themselves, but straight steps and change steps are not interchangeable with each other. However, a "straight + change" combination can be replaced with a "change + straight" combination.

8

As a leader you will need to communicate to your dance partner what kind of step you are leading. Your partner will commonly start a figure on the opposite foot (mirroring you), but occasionally both of you will start on the same foot, depending on what figures you are doing and what effect you are trying to achieve.

It should also be added that Lindy Hop is a forgiving dance and even if you mix up your feet (which tends to happen a lot initially) you always have a chance to fix it, usually by adding a quick extra step (without your partner noticing), or by pausing for a few seconds and then defaulting to a rock step at the beginning of the next 8-count section of the music. Jumping and landing on both feet is a crude but effective way to fix (or re-set) your footwork.

Aerial moves

There is a distinct group of Lindy Hop figures worth mentioning, namely the "aerials". These acrobatic figures include various leaps, flips and slides, and throwing your partner (or being thrown) in the air. As such, these figures carry a significant risk of injury. Since they are too dangerous for social dancing, they are mostly reserved for stage performances or competition dancing. Most social dancers will not be able to learn these figures, and social dance organizers will not allow them anyway for obvious safety reasons. Therefore these figures are not discussed in this book.

Building blocks of the dance

This chapter is the shortest in this book, but it is probably also the most important because it offers a structure for understanding and learning the dance.

Because Lindy Hop feeds from various sources and uses various rhythms and footwork, it can seem confusing to the initial observer or new student. To create order from chaos it is useful to classify various elements of the dance into a few meaningful categories.

Varied and enjoyable Lindy Hop dancing has five broad groups of basic components or building elements:

1. The common Lindy Hop steps and figures (including 6- and 8-count steps)

2. Charleston steps, including:

    a. Lindy Hop figures danced with Charleston footwork, or modified Charleston footwork

    b. Figures of the 1920s Classic Charleston and Breakaway dances

3. Footwork variations applied to the above figures

4. Break (or solo jazz) steps

5. Repetitive steps, checked steps and redirections

It is possible to dance the Lindy Hop using only the basic Lindy and Charleston steps, and you should do just that once you learn the basics. But eventually, to become a well-rounded dancer, one should gain a certain level of competence in all five areas. Only then will you be able to enjoy the improvisational nature of the dance to its full potential.

Learning the Lindy Hop

Learning from a book

Can one learn to dance from a book alone? No, one cannot any more than to learn to swim or to play tennis. Learning any skill, especially a complex social-physical skill like dancing has many aspects and several phases. It requires an intellectual understanding of the basic concepts and steps, preferably an understanding of the historical and social background, it requires observing demonstrations and receiving face-to-face instruction, and above all it requires persistent practice, both alone and with a variety of partners.

A book can help with the first aspect, and this can be a significant help. Going to group lessons knowing what to expect, recognizing what is being taught (and not taught), and better assessing your own progress are an advantage compared to facing it all without any prior understanding of what's coming at you. It can mean the difference between frustration and acceptance, between giving up and persevering, and ultimately between learning to dance or not.

Reading this book, taking lessons and going out to dance should go hand-in-hand. As you learn and practice more, the material in this book will also make more and more sense.

Flexible rules

Lindy Hop is a "street dance" (although it is generally danced indoors on a dance floor) which means that it has no written rules, no generally accepted standardization and no official body or society to decide in such matters. There is no official "technique book", like in ballroom dancing, that one could check or refer to. Lindy Hop does not have a standard set of steps or figures, and even many popular, commonly used figures have no generally accepted names.

When you learn any "rules" in Lindy Hop, whether in class or on the Internet, you need to remember in the back of your mind that these are the rules you will start breaking once you get the hang of the dance.

Having said this, every dance will have some commonly understood elements and there is a certain common set of basic moves and leads that most Lindy Hoppers learn wherever in the world they happen to live. This book explains those basic moves in some detail.

Certain steps go by various names in various countries or even in different parts of the same country. Often, group class instructors cannot put a name to the steps they teach. So when I named the figures described in this book I choose the names that seemed (to me) the most commonly used. It is likely that you will encounter them under some other names in a class or on the Internet. For certain steps, I could not find a name at all, so I just made one up. In any case, in social dancing steps are led, not discussed, and so the whole nomenclature eventually becomes irrelevant.

When learning a dance (or anything else), it is rewarding to go back to the original sources as much as possible. In the case of Lindy Hop this means a couple of things. One is old movies and movie clips containing dance scenes, typically from the 1930s or '40s. While these are amazing and instructive, they are often choreographed performances not representative of social dancing. There are exceptions however, showing scenes of actual social dancing, or even staged pieces that are suitable for social dancing.

Another rich source of information are books, such as the autobiography of Frankie Manning. These provide a vivid picture of the era when Lindy Hop was born (rather than descriptions of particular steps), and how the dance came to be what it is.

Lastly, one can find invaluable instructional videos from the 1980s and '90s by the then old Frankie Manning and other original Savoy dancers.

The steps covered in this book

The figures covered here are just a sampler but they are more than enough to provide a foundation that you can build on.

One can of course continue learning new steps, and no doubt you will. Learning new figures, however, can become a self-serving exercise. The essence of swing dancing is playfulness, style and improvisation. Dancing well what you know is more important than constantly learning new steps.

This book has no pictures, illustrations or foot charts, partly because they are not particularly useful, and partly because one can easily find these steps in a Lindy Hop class or in online videos. I will describe the mechanics of each step but without going into minute details.

Only steps that can be led and followed are included, and those figures (mini-choreographies) that the follower has to have memorized beforehand in order to perform it on cue are excluded.

Where a figure has both 6-count and 8-count versions, the version will be noted in brackets after the name of the figure ("6c" or "8c").

Each of these steps has numerous variations and several ways to start and exit them, other than those presented.

When indicating the direction of turns, the words "inside turn" and "outside turn" are frequently used. A quick Internet search reveals that there is complete confusion as to what these terms mean. In this book, an inside turn is where the leader's hand moves between (inside) the partners. An outside turn is the opposite.

Group classes

Group classes are useful entry points into the world of Lindy Hop, and they are good for learning the basic steps and the initial experience of dancing with many followers. You should take every group class offered where you live.

Local teachers of Lindy Hop tend to be nice people who do it out of love for the dance, and for this reason alone they deserve special appreciation. Without them, there would be no Lindy Hop. They are typically not professional dance instructors and do it part-time while having a day job.

But group classes also have their limitations. They tend to cover limited material, do not allow for much individual attention and don't have enough time to drill the steps. As a general rule, learning Lindy Hop in group classes will not be an overly structured experience. It is more like picking up bits and pieces as you go along. It will require patience and flexibility and, ideally, an advance overall understanding of the dance.

Getting into the details without explaining the big picture is a common shortcoming. This may be due either to the teacher's skill or "teacher's fatigue" that sets in when one has to explain the same thing to the 26th batch of beginners.

Because of the varied sources of Lindy Hop, classes can be downright confusing for the beginner. 8-count and 6-count steps, Charleston steps and jazz steps may be taught in a haphazard manner, leaving the beginner to wonder: "why are we doing this?"

Breaking down a figure to its individual steps and leading the class through it step-by-step, the teaching method common in almost all other dances, seems absent from Lindy Hop instruction. It is more likely: "We show it twice, really fast – now it's your turn!", which can be very difficult to follow. Consider repeating classes at least once to pick up what you missed on first exposure.

Dance instruction is a difficult art. Al Minns, one of the great Savoy dancers was remembered (in Norma Miller's book "Swingin' at the Savoy") by one of his students in the 1980s as a teacher who could not explain steps very well, kept miscounting the timing and often mixed up the men's and women's steps.

After explaining that Lindy Hop is a street dance without rules, some instructors can get pretty insistent about which of the non-existent rules you should follow. Various instructors will further insist on techniques that contradict each other. It is best to just follow each instructor's method in class and then to decide for yourself what works best for you.

As a practical matter, bring a bottle of water to classes, a folding fan if it is a hot day, and stay away from the loudspeakers. Chances are your instructor is unfamiliar with the hall's sound system, including the volume controls.

Finally, dancers in one community or geographic area tend to know each other and take the same classes, and so a certain location may develop a certain preferred style of dancing that differs from other locations in the same country or abroad.

It goes without saying that you should regularly go out and practice what you learned in class. It is also helpful to remember that when the Lindy Hop was born in the 1920s, there were no classes at all to learn it. Dancers learned new dances by watching others do it.

As such, group classes should have an important but limited place in your dance life, and you should not rely on them too heavily in learning the dance. The only place one can really learn to dance is on the social dance floor. Think of the classes as just a bonus, because ultimately it is up to you whether you will learn to dance or not.

Workshops and camps

Swing dance schools or dance clubs often organize workshops around a certain topic that can last over a couple of days, often crammed into a weekend.

Participating in Lindy Hop weekends, camps or other multi-day learning events is an excellent way to give your dancing a much needed push. They are fun, they expose you to other teachers than your regular ones and give you a confidence boost by making you feel that you are part of the "community".

The best time to attend workshops is after taking the beginner and intermediate level group classes available, and practicing what you learned by going to social dances.

If you live in or near a major urban centre you should definitely take the opportunities conveniently offered locally. Otherwise, participating in these events requires some travel. If you want to attend an event in another part of the country or abroad, you may plan your next vacation around it.

There is also a large selection of Lindy Hop videos available online. These are great for identifying steps, figuring out the details of steps taught in class, and also to see how different people dance certain figures. The quality of these videos varies widely but one can learn something from most, including old footage of social dancing from the 1930s and 40s.

Practicing

If there is one secret to learning the Lindy Hop, it is the same secret that applies to learning any other skill: consistent and persistent practice. This mainly means two things: practicing alone and going to social dances as often as you can.

You definitely should practice alone. The partner connection will be missing, but it is a good way to observe and study a figure undisturbed. Free up some floor space at home, and do that figure slowly, step by step, paying attention to what your feet, arms, hands, body and head are doing, and where your follower would be at any point in time. Allow your body to gradually get used to the sequence of muscle movements that make up a figure. Do it again and again, increasingly faster. Repeat it 50 or 100 times, until you can do it at any time without paying attention. Practice transitions between figures, practice getting into figures and exiting figures. Study and practice how to start and end a dance.

You should also go out and dance while you practice at home. The social dance floor is the best teacher. Not going to social dances until you are sure that you have all the steps nailed down guarantees that you will never learn to dance.

You need to know and accept that going to social dances while you still learn to dance also guarantees that you will fail a lot. Initially, it can be frustrating having to dance and practice simple and boring figures, and failing even at that. Don't worry about it. Failure is the price of success, and trying and failing is the only way to learn, so the best option is to embrace failing as part of the process that leads to success.

So swallow your pride and forge ahead. There is no other way. Keep practicing until it is second nature, until you cannot get it wrong anymore.

Private lessons

Taking private lessons with a local Lindy Hop instructor can be a good ways to increase your dance skills. What results you get out of private lessons depends on the effort you put into them. You have to know your objectives with taking the classes and work to achieve them.

Just as with Lindy workshops and camps, taking private lessons is most useful in the "mid-range" of your development. This is the level where you are most likely to get stuck. Some personal attention and individual feedback can give you a "push" and help you move along.

Taking private lessons earlier than this is not cost effective, and later, when you have already mastered the dance, you will not need them anymore.

At this "mid-range" of your development, private lessons can be useful in a number of areas.

- You can gain the experience of dancing with a good dancer.
- The instructor will observe you and point out the areas where you need improvement.
- You can obtain instruction and practice in "specialty" areas not covered by group classes, such as dancing to slow and fast music
- You can ask any questions you have about learning and social dancing.
- It will likely improve your general confidence in dancing.

To find an instructor who offers private lessons, ask the teachers in your group classes and/or your classmates. Since your teachers will likely be amateurs who do this part-time, the cost should not be prohibitive.

There is no need to go overboard with private lessons. Budget for five lessons, then take a break and practice what you learned. Let it sink in. After a few months, you can assess where your weak points are and whether there is anything new you want to learn. Then you may take a few more lessons to cover those areas.

Have a plan and an agenda for each private lesson. Write down your questions well before each lesson, otherwise you will forget to ask them. At the same time be flexible and remain open to your instructor's suggestions because she will probably notice things that you never even thought about.

Taking private lessons can have logistical challenges, most importantly the physical space for the lesson. Your instructor may not be able to secure a practice room with proper dance floor, so she may ask you to come up with your own space. Depending on the place you find, the floor can range from hard wood to tile to carpet, each with its own challenges. Your instructor should bring her music, typically stored on her phone. If a sound system is not available, the phone's speaker should be adequate for practice. Plug in the phone so the battery won't die halfway through the lesson.

Have pen and paper ready during the lesson and write down what was covered that day, anything important that you learned, and every piece of advice received from your instructor. In-between lessons review and practice what you learned.

Remember that private lessons are not a replacement for group classes or social dancing so don't use them as a cop-out.

Dance competitions

Dance competitions are a curious phenomenon for those who dance for the joy of dancing, and not to be better than someone else.

Others like the excitement and the spotlight, like to participate in the preparations and enjoy meeting fellow dancers from other communities, or they are semi-professional teachers who figure that winning a competition will attract more students or more teaching invitations.

Dance competitions, if not taken seriously, can be used to motivate yourself to stretch a little and to get to know who is who in your dance community.

Do I need a partner?

Perhaps you are wondering whether having a steady dance partner would be helpful in learning to dance. While with other dances, such as ballroom or Argentine Tango, this can be a real dilemma, with Lindy Hop it is generally not.

If you have a dance partner who you like to dance and practice with, that is fine but you will definitely not feel left out if you go to a class or dance alone. Lindy Hop instructors will generally rotate the students in class, and swing social dance events tend to be friendly and informal where most everyone is approachable and willing to dance with anyone.

Having a steady dance partner who you can practice with and grow together has some advantages. She will be familiar with your lead and therefore know how to follow it, which can be satisfying. On the other hand, your ability to lead new partners will diminish, and you will miss out on the social aspect of dancing.

Clothing

When dancing Lindy Hop, your most important piece of clothing will be your shoes. You need comfortable, well-fitting, flexible shoes with a sole that is not sticky but not too slippery either. Avoid rubber soles but certain hard man-made soles work well. Leather soled dress shoes are generally fine for dancing. There are purpose-built, vintage inspired swing dance shoes on the market in the style of the 1930s and '40s, however they are expensive and not necessary for good dancing.

An inexpensive and practical solution is to take a comfortable pair of old street shoes, clean and wash the sole, and glue a thin layer of suede leather on it, including the heels. Sheets of suede leather can be purchased at crafts stores and strong shoe glue is available at any hardware store. After dancing, clean off the suede sole with a cheap nail brush set aside for that purpose, and occasionally brush it up with a wire brush to prevent it from becoming compacted. If the suede wears out (which takes a long time) you can simply replace it or glue a new layer on top of the old. If you don't feel up to the task, ask a cobbler to do it for you.

In an emergency, you can fix your sticky shoes by adding some duct tape to the sole.

The rest of your clothing should be light and should not restrict your movement. Ideal are light cotton or linen pants with a comfortable cut. Similarly, shirts should be light and made of a fabric that absorbs moisture. If you dance for any length of time, you will be sweating but you don't necessarily want it to show. Moisture absorbing polyester shirts, T-shirts or golf shirts are usually great and some of them are quite stylish.

It is a good idea to bring a spare shirt to a dance. When you get soaked, go to the rest room and change into the spare.

Old photos of the Savoy Ballroom invariably show dancers dressed up nicely. This does not necessarily have much to do with Lindy Hop; people just used have more style back then. Men without a coat and tie were often not allowed in.

These days most swing dancers dress casually when they go out to dance, although some do dress up better. Others like to wear a variety of 1930s to 1950s attire which is cool and certainly adds to the fun.

Safety

Dancing is vigorous physical activity and it puts serious stress on the body. Dance at your own risk, and make sure that you are suitably fit before you start. If you have any doubts, ask your doctor for advice.

You should warm up before practice, classes or dances. Warming up is important before any physical activity and dancing is no exception.

Before attempting any step or figure, make sure that you can execute them without accidents or injuries to you, your partner or anyone else.

Two points specifically are worth mentioning: 1) shoulders are delicate, and 2) knees are not designed to last forever.

The risk of injury to shoulder joints applies mostly to followers. If you notice that your follower is weak, older or holds her arms at dangerous angles, be extra gentle with her.

The knee is one of the common body parts to be injured and Lindy Hop is very demanding on the knees. It involves most of the typical risk factors for the knee: over-use, twisting, bending and sudden changes in direction, particularly in some of the jazz or break steps.

Naturally, the older the dancer the more acute the potential problems of the knee. Young people tend to think that they will live forever and their body parts can take any abuse without consequences. This is, however not so. You may forget what you did to your knees, but your knees will remind you one day.

There are a few simple things you can do to protect your knees. First, wear shoes with soles suitable for dancing (avoid sticky rubber soles) and dance on proper dance surfaces. Second, keep your knees under you or slightly in front of you. Third, make sure that your knee and toes always point into the same direction. It doesn't matter how many figures you know if you are unable to walk.

You should also carry a water bottle and drink frequently to avoid dehydration, and stay away from the loudspeakers to protect your hearing.

Posture and connection

Posture

Every dance has a certain basic posture or "poise" that is most efficient for that particular dance. The best posture is the one that accommodates the dynamic movements of the dancing couple.

Lindy Hop is an energetic, fast-paced dance. Dancers maintain a relaxed but active, grounded stance that allows the legs to move quickly in any direction. Try to be low in the lower part of your body, knees flexed, muscles relaxed, and more upright in your upper body.

Pulsing

Swing music has a clear rhythm, and allowing your body to "pulse" with the rhythm keeps you in sync both with the music and your dance partner. Pulsing is moving your body down and up to the rhythm of the music. It is not bouncing on your toes, rather it is a downward pulsing with relaxed knees.

Pulsing is your inner metronome, and a close relative to clapping to the music. It is, by the way, okay to clap to the music before you start a dance, or even during a dance when you are separated from your partner and doing break steps.

With slower music the pulse will be deeper. With fast music the pulse necessarily will be shallower as there is not enough time for the body to move down and up so quickly. But pulsing should never cease completely. You should be able to keep up the pulsing when the music gets faster. Practice it alone, just pulsing without dancing, to various pieces of swing music of increasing tempo.

When using Charleston steps, the pulse is a little different because Charleston is danced in a more upright position, and you spend more time on the ball of your feet. The pulsing in Charleston has a more bouncy feel to it.

Connection and positions

The connection between the two dancers and their relative position changes constantly during the dance.

Two common positions relative to each other are the open position and the closed position. In open position, the dancers stand apart and have only hand contact, or they may not be touching at all. In closed position, the partners stand close to each other, the leader rests his right hand on the follower's back and takes the follower's right hand with his left hand. Closed position can be side-by-side or facing each other.

There are other positions including the cuddle (sweetheart) and the tandem (one dancer behind the other) positions.

Stand beside the follower, to her left, and put your right hand around her waist. She will put her left arm on top of your right shoulder. Take her right hand with your left hand and let your hands hang loosely in front of you. You are now in a side-by-side closed position. You can turn more toward each other and it is still a closed position. While dancing in closed position, your right hand will move naturally between the follower's waist and the middle of her back throughout the dance, depending on your distance and relative position to each other.

Now stand in front of your follower facing her, step back a little, take her right hand with your left hand and let your right hand hang at your side. You are now in an open position. If you take right-to-right handhold or double handhold, it is still an open position.

Handhold

When you take the follower's hand, avoid grabbing or clutching it or putting your thumb on top of her hand. Rather, offer your three middle fingers as a hook that she can use to hook her fingers into. Any tension should be in your fingers, not in your arm.

The handhold can be:

- left-to-right (your left hand to her right hand, the most common handhold)
- right-to-right (cross-hold or handshake)
- double handhold (both hands holding her opposing hands as she is facing you)
- double cross-hold (you cross your hands, left over right, and take her opposing hands as she is facing you)
- right-to-left and left-to-left handholds are rarely used

In certain figures you will move toward each other, pressing your hands against the follower's and creating a push or compression between your hands. The position of the hands will have to accommodate this, connecting either palm-to-palm or palm-to-fist.

Use of the arms

In an open position, your free arm(s) should swing naturally in opposition to your foot on the same side and in agreement with the other foot. This is not different from natural body movement when briskly walking or running.

Basic 8-count steps

Some of the basic figures described in this and the following chapter are the core steps of Lindy Hop. These are typically taught in introductory Lindy Hop classes and they are indispensable for social dancing.

The basic rhythm of 8-count figures is "1-2-3&4-5-6-7&8", and the basic footwork pattern is "rock-step-triple-step-step-step-triple-step". Drill this pattern into muscle memory and remember to keep pulsing.

Closed Basic and Gliding

The Closed Basic is really just the basic 8-count Lindy footwork: "rock-step-triple-step-step-step-triple-step" done in side-by-side closed position, more or less in one place. Keep a relaxed connection and keep pulsing.

The rock step, also known as "back & replace", is a ubiquitous step in Lindy Hop and serves as the opening or anchor step of many figures. It consist of taking a back step on one foot (left for the lead, right for the follow) and then replacing (shifting back) the body weight to the other foot.

You can gradually turn left or right and even move around the dance floor with your partner while doing the Closed Basic, taking small steps into the direction of your choice, instead of doing the whole thing in one place. This moving around is called Gliding. It is a useful "warm-up" to do when you start a dance with a stranger, so that you can get used to moving together and ease into a common rhythm or pulse. It is also useful for moving to another location on the dance floor if your current location is problematic. In an emergency, or when dancing with an absolute beginner, Gliding can take you through a song without anyone noticing.

Flip Flop

Start in a side-by-side closed position and let go of the follower's right hand, keeping your left hand free. Do a rock step, then triple-step forward while turning towards your partner and leading her to do the same. Continue turning and by the end of the triple step both of you will have made a half turn and be in a side-by-side closed position facing the opposite direction. She will now be on your left. Do a rock step (this time with your right foot) and triple-step back to your starting position in the same fashion, again turning 180 towards each other.

Instead of flip-flopping forward and back, you can rock-step and then flip (triple-step) your partner from your right side across in front of you to your left side while you triple-step in one place, then flop her back to your right side (aka "Toss Across"). Or you can flip yourself from her left side to her right side and back while letting her stay in one place.

You can vary the Flip-Flop by doing it variously forward and back, left or right, or alternating between flipping your partner and yourself.

This simple step (and the next two, which are also very simple) should not be underestimated. When practiced in class as a beginner routine, they may seem boring, but they can be used to good effect in social dancing, mixed with other steps.

He-Goes-She-Goes

This step starts from a closed, side-by-side position. You will triple-step out and turn 180 to the right to face your follower, then triple-step back to her side. She will then in turn do the same. In more detail:

He Goes: Do a rock step on 1-2, then triple-step in front of her on 3&4 making a half turn to right to face her while she stays in place. Now do a rock step on 5-6 leading her into a forward rock step, and then triple-step back to your original position at her side on 7&8.

She Goes: Do a rock step on 1-2, then lead her to turn 180 left as she triple-steps in front of you on 3&4. Now do a forward rock step on 5-6 leading her into a back rock step, then lead her to triple-step back to your right side in closed position on 7&8.

Keep holding her right hand with your left hand and keep your right hand on her back throughout.

Promenade

The Promenade is danced on a slot on the dance floor back and forth.

It starts like a He Goes or a She Goes, but 5-6 will not be a rock-step to check the movement. Instead, 5-6 will be walking steps to continue the movement along the slot. For the lead, 5-6 will be two forward steps on a She Goes, and two back steps on a He Goes. The figure is completed just like a He-Goes-She-Goes, and the party travelling forward will triple-step to the other party's side into closed position on 7&8.

For example: Do a rock-step and triple-step her out to face you, walk two steps forward with her, and triple-step to her side. Now do another rock-step, triple-step out to face her, walk two steps backward with her, and triple-step her back to your side.

Texas Tommy

Also known as "Handshake behind the Back" or "Apache Turn". Start from open position facing each other, do a rock step, then triple-step towards each other without turning much.

As you approach, on 3&4 gently put your left hand around her at waist level while still holding her right hand. Place her hand, palm out, on her lower back. Keep your left hand low and relaxed, and the handhold loose, to avoid straining her arm. Your left hand is now holding her right hand behind her back. Put your right hand around her as well, and pass her hand from your left hand to your right hand. Often it will be easier to catch her wrist with your right hand and let her hand slide into yours. Keep your hands low. You are now in a right-to-right ("handshake") handhold, albeit behind her back.

On 5-6 both of you will turn around each other to "untangle" her hand (half right turn for you and 1.5 right turn for her), and then back away from each other on the last triple-step, effectively trading places.

The Texas Tommy is a simple but great-looking move. It can be added as a variation to other steps, like the Swingout, as well.

Notice that you end the figure with a R2R cross handhold, so your next step should be something that starts with this handhold.

Tuck Turn (8c)

Also called "Tuck-in Turn".

Start from a side-by-side closed position. Do a rock step on 1-2. On the first triple step (3&4) lead the follower to step in front of you, turn and face you, and raise your left hand at the same time. On 5-6 lead an outside (right) turn with your left hand and slowly bring your hand down at the end of 6. On the second triple step (7&8) you will already be facing each other again.

Alternatively, on the first triple step send out the follower to turn and face you without raising your left hand. Use 5-6 to wind up the turn by moving your left hand to the right at waist level. Now lead the tuck turn with a big upward circle of your left hand on 7&8.

Double Tuck Turn (8c)

This is the same as the Tuck Turn except you will lead the follower into two continuous turns: one on 5-6 and the second on 7&8.

You can end the figure in open position, face-to-face, or you can turn to left and triple-step to her side on 7&8, put your right hand around her waist and end in closed position.

Tuck Turn Push-Around (8c)

Start from a side-by-side closed position. Do a rock step on 1-2. On the first triple step lead the follower to turn and face you in a slightly offset position to right, and at the same time raise your left hand indicating an upcoming turn.

On 5-6 lead her into a tuck turn, and then on 7&8 continue guiding her, with your right hand on her, back to move around you clockwise. Keep your left hand over your head with a loose connection (fingers on fingers) and lower it after she has progressed around you. Stay in one place throughout, facing your original direction.

It is unlikely that she will be able to do a complete circle around you. By the second triple-step she will be somewhere on your left side. You can use this position to do some side-by-side break steps, or you can turn to your left to face her in open position, ready for the next step.

Change of Places (8c)

This is an 8-count underarm pass starting from face-to-face open position.

Do a rock-step (1-2), then raise your left hand to indicate the upcoming turn (3&4). Lead the follower into an underarm left turn ("inside turn") passing in front of you from left to right (5-6). Keep up your left hand on 5-6 (step-step) to indicate that it is an 8-count move and bring it down after 6 to complete the turn. On the last triple-step (7&8), you will be facing each other again.

During the figure, turn gradually to right and move to the left in order to "change places" with her.

Alternatively, lead the underarm turn on 3&4, and use 5-6 to "wind her up" again by moving your left hand to your right at waist level. Now lead a right turn (opposite to the first turn) with a wide upward circular motion of your left hand on 7&8.

Cuddle (8c)

Start from open position, double handhold, facing each other. Do a rock step extending your arms slightly so that she also does a rock step, then lead her with your left hand into an inside underarm turn (left turn) on the first triple step (3&4). Lower your left hand at the end of the triple step while maintaining double handhold.

At this point she will be next to you on your right side, facing the same direction. You will hold her left hand with your right hand around her waist in a cuddle or "sweetheart" position.

Do another rock step together (5-6), then on the second triple step lead her back the way she came, raising your left hand again and letting her back out, turning under your arm. This will "untangle" the cuddle and you will both end up in your starting positions.

Swingout

The Swingout originated from the Breakaway and it is a signature figure of Lindy Hop. It is an 8-count move. It can start from either a closed or open position and ends in an open position, the partners having made a full turn around each other.

When starting from open position, facing each other, with normal L2R handhold, the initial rock step creates a stretch between the partners. On the first triple step (3&4) the partners use this stretch to move towards each other with strong momentum, turning a quarter to right and passing by each other face-to-face in close proximity. Put your right hand on her back as you pass her and continue turning right. On 4, check the momentum of the turn with your knees slightly bent and your right hand on her back, again resulting in a good stretch. You now face each other in a face-to-face closed position, both having made a half turn.

The stretch of step 4 will give her enough momentum to start moving forward on 5-6 and pass by you again while you get out of her way. This is referred to as "swinging her out". There is no need to pull her in order to swing her out. However, when dancing with a beginner, a gentle pull on 5 may be necessary to guide her along.

On 5-6, both of you will do another half turn to the right, completing a 360. On 7&8, triple-step back to where you started from, more or less. Do not end up too far from your partner at the end of the Swingout.

The can turn either sooner or later on the exit – this partly depends on the lead but also on her styling. If she turns to face the lead sooner (on 5 or 6), she will exit the Swingout "backward", but if she only turns at the very end (7&8), she will exit "forward". To lead a "backward" exit, hold on to her back longer (i.e. keep her in closed position longer). If you let go of her back soon, she can then choose whether to exit backward or forward.

You have a few options for choosing your step on 5. You can step straight back, you can step diagonally across behind your left foot, or you can step diagonally across in front of your left foot. Each can work. Your job is to get out of your partner's way while making another half turn to the right. If on 4 you are already in an offset position (so that she is slightly to your right), then you can step straight back and she will still be able to pass by you narrowly as you both turn. If on 4 you are facing her square, then you will have to step out of her way. Instructors tend to have their favourite version, so just do what they say, and then see what works best for you.

It is also possible to do the Swingout from a side-by-side closed position. Start with a rock step and use the first triple step to get in front of your partner facing her ("He Goes"), with your right hand on her back and your knees slightly bent, creating the necessary stretch on 4. From here, proceeds with the exit as explained.

Keep your left hand low throughout the Swingout and do not raise it unless you are preparing to insert an underarm turn.

The Swingout is typically a linear figure. The follower tends to travel more than the leader, moving back and forth along a straight line, and swinging around the leader who stays closer to the centre of the action, focusing on swinging her out and then getting out of her way. However, the step can be danced underturned, overturned, or in a more circular manner, depending on the dancers' style and preferences and the available space on the dance floor.

A common footwork variation for the follower is to do swivels (twist steps) on 8-1-2, replacing the basic rock step. These swivels have been a characteristic feature of the dance since the 1930s.

Swingout with Turns

You can vary the Swingout so that the follower performs an inside (left) or outside (right) turn on the second, exit half of the Swingout ("back end").

You can also lead an inside or outside turn on the first, entry half ("front end") if you start from an open position.

The inside turn is only a half turn for the follower (she turns left instead of right) but the outside turn is a one-and-a-half turn, therefore it is far more difficult for her to do.

1/ Back-end (exit) turns of the follower

When you lead an inside turn on the back end, raise your left hand in front of you and above your forehead, palm out, by the end of the first triple step (beat 4) to indicate that an inside turn is coming on 5-6. On the exit she will now make a half turn to left under your arm, instead of the usual half turn to right. Most of her turn will happen on 6. Bring your hand down before the last triple step.

When you lead an outside turn on the back end, again raise your left hand by the end of the first triple step (beat 4), but this time somewhat to your left, to indicate that an outside turn is coming on 5-6 and to give her space to pass under your arm. This time she will make a full right turn on top of the usual half turn. Bring your hand down after 6 to lead her to face you again.

The outside turn on the exit can also be led "hands-free", which means that you initiate an outside free spin with your right hand on her back, let go of her hand and catch it again when her turn is completed. This time you don't need to raise your left hand as you are not using it to lead the turn.

Lastly, you can lead the outside turn with a Texas Tommy, where you pass the follower's right hand from your left hand into your right hand behind her back on 3&4. Keep your left hand low and relaxed, and bring her right hand out to the side a bit before sliding it behind her back close to her body. Do not grab and pull her hand with your right hand, rather let her complete her turn and let her hand naturally slide into yours. This move ends with a R2R handshake handhold which can be used to lead certain steps (for example a Right Side Pass or an American Turn).

2/ Front-end (entrance) turns

The follower's turns on the first, entrance half of the Swingout are trickier for the leader because he has to catch a turning follower and be in Swingout position on 4.

3/ Leader's turns

The follower is not the only one who can turn during the Swingout. You can insert a turn of your own on the back-end of the Swingout (not on the front end, because then you need to focus on catching your follower on 4).

On the exit, instead of the usual half-turn to your right, make a half-turn to left under your own arm. This works fine whether you lead the follower into an exit with an inside or outside turn, or without a turn.

Alternatively, do a full free spin to right on 6 while leading an outside free turn for the follower.

Lindy Circle

The Lindy Circle is similar to the Swingout except you do not swing out your partner on the second 4 beats. Instead, keep her in closed position and finish the figure that way. The Lindy Circle, like the Swingout can start from an open or closed position, but it always ends in closed position. 5-6 is a turning step-step, rather than a rock step.

When it starts from an open position, the Lindy Circle is sometimes referred to as a "Bring-In". You can "bring her in" leading an inside or outside turn with your left hand over her head, or if you happen to start with a right-to-right handhold you can lead her into a left turn by drawing your right hand in and across to the right. Keep holding her hand and wrap your right arm around her waist as you bring her in.

On the last triple step the couple could travel backwards (making sure not to bump into anyone behind them) to break the circularity of the movement.

To keep the circularity, continue rotating on the last triple step. The choice will depend mainly on the nature of your intended next figure.

Frisbee (8c)

Start from open position. When doing the rock-step, swing your left hand out to left on 1 and let it drop down on 2. Using this momentum, turn a quarter to right and triple forward (3&4). This will serve to wind up both of you for the upcoming turn.

Now lead a full outside turn for both of you on 5-6 while moving to your right (left turn for you and a right turn for her, mirroring each other). Re-connect on 7&8 in an open position, facing each other.

You can also overturn at the end, put your right arm around her and re-connect in a side-by-side closed position.

The Frisbee is a natural addition to the Double Tuck Turn as it continues the ending motion of that figure.

Boomerang

Also referred to as "Lock Whip" or "Basket". You will lead her to move forward and pass you on your right side, check her, and lead her to back out on your other side. She will face one direction throughout.

Start from an open position with double handhold. Do a rock step. On 3, step to the left to get out of her way and lead her to triple-step forward on a straight line under your left arm. Keep the double handhold. Let her pass on your right and turn right 180 with her. On 4, step behind her. You are still holding both of her hands while her arms are crossed in front of her. Stop or "check" her forward movement gently on 4.

Now lead her to step (boomerang) back on a straight line without turning (5-6). You will step left again to get out of her way, and continue turning to right after her. On the last triple step (7&8), let go of your right hand as you complete the step facing her in your starting position.

During this figure, she will move on a straight path forward and backward without turning, while you turn 360 to your right in a small circle.

It is possible to lead the Boomerang with normal left-to-right handhold, instead of double handhold, but be aware that the follower will likely anticipate a Change of Places, so keep your left arm loose and make sure not to lead her to turn. She should move forward on a straight line and not turn. Step aside and out of her way on the first triple step. When she has passed you, grab her right hip with your free right hand as soon as you can (before the end of the first triple step) to check her and send her back on 5-6. This version is less precisely controlled because you don't have the double handhold that keeps her in lock, so she is less likely to travel on a straight path forward and back. There is a risk that she will turn on her own no matter what you lead.

Basic 6-count steps

The basic design and rhythm of these figures have much in common with the ballroom dances Jive and East Coast Swing and can be danced at events that cater to those dances.

The basic rhythm of 6-count figures is 1-2-3&4-5&6, and the basic step pattern is "rock-step-triple-step-triple-step".

Closed and Open Basic

The basic 6-count step for the leader consists of a rock step, a triple-step to the left and a triple-step to the right, in closed or open position.

6-count Circle

The Basic can be varied by rotating to the left or to the right.

If you want to turn right, then after the rock step do 3&4 forward and turning right, and then 5&6 backward and still turning right.

If you want to turn left, do the rock step slightly across and behind your right foot, setting up the left turning motion. Then do 3&4 more or less in one place and 5&6 forward and to the right, continuously turning left and leading her around you.

Sendout

The Sendout (also called "Throwout") is leading (or sending out) your follower from a closed, side-by-side position into an open, face-to-face position while doing the basic 6-count footwork.

Do a rock step, then slightly lean forward on the first triple step and gently guide her forward. She will swivel to left on 5 and do the second triple step facing you in an open position.

You can also do a forward rock step (aka "opposition break") on 1-2 (while she does a regular rock step) go give her a good stretch in preparation for the send-out.

Rollout

This is a Sendout variation, adding an inside (left) turn for the follower on 3&4.

On 1-2, do a forward rock step (opposition break) while she does a regular rock step. Turn her to right on 1 (wind her up for the turn), then turn her left on 2 while raising your left hand, and send her out ("roll her out") with a full left spin on 3&4. Lead the spin with a clockwise circular motion of your left hand over her head.

On the second triple step (5&6) she will have already finished her turn and be in an open position facing you.

Pop Turn

This is a Rollout led without using your left hand. Use your right hand around the follower's waist to lead her into an inside (left) free spin with a motion of your wrist.

Like every free turn, this is an opportunity to switch to another handhold at the end.

Tuck Turn (6c)

This is a shorter version of the 8-count Tuck Turn.

Start from a side-by-side closed position. Do a rock step on 1-2. On the first triple step lead the follower to step in front of you, turn and face you, and raise your left hand at the same time. On 5&6 lead an outside (right) underarm turn with your left hand and bring your hand down quickly on 6.

You can also lead the Tuck Turn as a free spin, without using your left hand, leading with your right arm only, and catch her hand when she completed her turn. This is an opportunity to switch handholds if your next move requires a "handshake" handhold.

To give the Tuck Turn a stronger momentum, replace the rock step with a front rock step (opposition break) while she does a regular rock step. This can be particularly effective if the Tuck Turn follows a circular figure, such as a Lindy Circle.

You will lead the 6-count Tuck Turn more firmly and quickly than the 8-count version. The lead for the 8-count Tuck Turn is more relaxed. This is how the follower can tell the difference.

American Turn

This is somewhat similar to the Tuck Turn but it is led from an open, face to face position and uses a R2R handhold.

Start from open position, facing each other, right-to-right "handshake" handhold. Do a rock step. On the first triple-step (3&4), move your right hand to your right at waist level to turn her out and wind her up, then let her hand compress against yours (4) to give her the leverage for her upcoming turn. On 5&6 lead an underarm right turn with a wide circular motion of your right hand, starting low, then across and up to the left and over her head.

The American Turn can also be led as free turn. Compress your right hand against hers on 4 and then give her a push to send her into a free right spin on 5&6.

Change of Places (6c)

This is a shorter version of the 8-count Change of Places. It is a 6-count underarm pass starting from face-to-face open position.

Do a rock step lifting your left hand on 2. On 3&4, lead the follower into an inside (left) turn passing in front of you from left to right. Bring your hand down on 4. On 5&6, you will be facing each other again.

During 3&4-5&6, turn gradually to right and move to left in order to "change places" with the follower by the end of the move.

Make the Change of Places more interesting by keeping your left hand up and doing a left turn yourself (under your own left arm) on 5&6, immediately after her turn.

Generally speaking, it will not always be up to you whether a figure turns out 6-count or 8-count (or something else). You may intend to lead a 6-count Change of Places, but if the follower decides that she wants to do some jazz steps and turn it into an 8-count (or longer) figure, you just have to go along and accommodate it. Do some additional footwork and move on to the next step when she is ready.

Right Side Pass

This is similar to the Change of Places except it starts from a right-to-right handhold and it is a free turn for the follower.

After the rock step, lead her into a free left spin by pulling her right hand in a U-shape across in front of you and letting go of her hand while she commences her turn (3&4). Catch her hand again (with your left or right hand) after she completed a full turn, and do the second triple step in open position facing each other (5&6).

44

You can add some variety by doing a free right turn on your own while she does her left turn (3&4) and face her again on 5&6.

This step can be added to a figure that ends with a handshake handhold (like the Texas Tommy) if you want to switch back to regular handhold.

Belt Turn

Also known as Belt Slide. For a change, this is your turn, not the follower's turn. It starts from a standard (left-to-right) handhold in open position, facing each other.

Do a rock step (1-2). On the first triple step, lead the follower to pass you on your right side without turning while you make a full left turn (3&4). Let go of her hand as you start turning and let it wrap around you and slide along your waist (belt) as you continue turning. Lift your right hand a little to keep it out of her way.

When you completed your turn, grab her hand either with your left or right hand (or both hands for a double handhold), depending on what move you want to do next. Do the second triple step in open position, facing each other (5&6).

Cuddle (6c)

This is similar to the 8-count Cuddle, and it starts from an open, face-to-face position with double handhold. It has a shorter version and a longer version.

On the short version, after the rock step you lead her into a cuddle on 3&4, and lead her back out right away on 5&6. Your first triple step will be slightly forward, the second slightly backward.

The longer version needs two 6-count cycles to complete. You pull her into the cuddle on the first cycle, and send out on the second cycle as follows.

Lead her into the cuddle on 3&4, moving slightly forward on the triple step, then do the second triple step (5&6) together in cuddle position, moving slightly backwards. This completes the first 6 counts. From here, do the next rock step together, still in cuddle position, then lead her out of the cuddle on 3&4. The last triple step (5&6) will already be in open position facing each other. You can let go of your right hand at this time.

Overhead Loop

Also known as "Miami Special". This is an elegant way to switch from cross handhold to a normal handhold.

Start from open position with a right-to-right "handshake" handhold. Do a rock step (1&2).

On the first triple-step, lead (with your right hand) a Change of Places with an underarm turn. As she does her underarm turn, step forward and turn to right to get side-by-side with her (she is on your left). Keep your right hand up, loop it over your head and place her right hand on your left shoulder. All this happens on 3&4.

On 5&6, triple-step away from each other, moving sideways (you to right, she to left). Let go of your right hand, and let her hand slide down on your left shoulder and arm into your left hand (5&6).

Frisbee (6c)

This is a shorter version of the 8-count Frisbee, and the turn will be into the opposite direction.

Start from open position, normal handhold. Do a rock-step sideways, stepping to left rather than back (1-2). Swing your left hand out to left on 1 and let it drop back on 2. This will serve to wind up both of you for the upcoming turn.

Using this momentum, lead a full inside turn for both of you on the first triple-step (3&4) while moving to your right (right turn for you and a left turn for her, mirroring each other). Reconnect for the last triple-step in an open position, facing each other (5&6).

Use your whole body, not just your arm to lead this figure.

Basic Lindy Charleston steps

When Lindy dancers talk about "Charleston steps" or "Charleston footwork", this is generally not a reference to the early 1920s Classic Charleston dance (which is, by the way, a fun dance). Rather, what is meant is a modified, "Charleston-looking" footwork adapted to and incorporated into Lindy Hop in the 1930s.

When the music gets faster, it becomes onerous to do very fast triple steps. Since the Charleston footwork replaces the triple step with a "kick-step" or a "groove step" (both of which represent one step instead of three), it is much better suited to fast music.

Kick-step

The "kick-step" is a characteristic feature of Charleston figures. While the rhythm of a triple-step is "1&2", in the kick-step the "1&" is replaced by a small kick in the air.

The "kicking" is done from the knee, not from the hip. It is more like letting your lower leg swing out on its own than an active kick. It is more of a flick than a kick, the heel leading, not the toes. The faster the music, the smaller the kick.

Both triple-step and kick-step are interchangeable "change steps" as each involves an odd number of weight changes: 3 on the triple-step versus 1 on the kick-step. As such, the kick-step is not limited to Charleston figures. It is a versatile footwork variation often used in Lindy to replace triple-steps for styling purposes. You can practice this by picking any Lindy figure and see how you can replace triple-steps with kick-steps.

Groove walk

The "groove step" or "groove walk" is the lazy man's kick-step. "Kick-step" is replaced with one single step done "heel-toe" when going forward or "toe-heel" when going backward. Groove steps are really just rhythmic single steps. You can replace kick-steps with groove walk if the music gets faster or when your energy level gets lower.

It is important to keep up your pulsing when doing kick steps or groove walk in order to feel the rhythm of the music and to maintain the character of the dance.

Charleston footwork patterns

There are several common Charleston footwork patterns used in Lindy Hop and they are more varied and complex than the basic Lindy Hop footwork.

When you use Charleston footwork, you need to know which pattern fits your intended figure. I will call the most commonly used Charleston patterns C1, C2, C3 and C4 as described below. This is not a standard classification, I just find it useful for getting a better grip on the Charleston variations.

- C1 (8c): tap-&-step-&-tap-&-step-&
  - This is the typical step pattern of the 1920s Classic Charleston
- C2 (8c): rock-step-kick-step-rock-step-kick-step
  - This is the Charleston version of the basic 8-count Lindy footwork
- C3 (8c): rock-step-kick-step-kick-&-kick-step
  - This is the 1930s "Charleston for Lindy" footwork
- C4 (6c): rock-step-kick-step-kick-step
  - This is the Charleston version of the basic 6-count Lindy footwork

This may seem complicated and somewhat contrived, but it only reflects the reality of the varied Charleston footwork options.

As you can see, for 8-count figures there are several Charleston footwork patterns, but with 6-count figures the Charleston footwork is always the same (C4).

Depending on the figure, Charleston footwork can be further varied (for example to involve multiple kick-steps or multiple kick-&-kick-steps).

This chapter includes both 6- and 8-count Charleston figures. For each step, I will indicate which Charleston footwork pattern is to be used or add further explanation where the footwork differs. For example "8c-C3" means that the step is an 8-count step and the C3 (typical Charleston for Lindy) footwork is to be used.

Charleston Basic (8c-C3)

This is typically the first figure you learn when getting into Lindy Charleston. It is also incorporated in Tandem Charleston and many other figures.

It is often danced side-by-side, your right arm around the follower's waist, similar to a closed position but letting go of the handhold.

The footwork is: rock step (1-2), kick-step (left forward, 3-4), kick& (right forward, 5-6) kick-step (right back, 7-8).

Notice that 5 is a kick forward with RF and 7 is a kick back with RF, keeping your RF in the air on 6 (so your RF is in the air for 3 beats).

Jig Kicks (6c-C4)

This is a 6-count step, so the footwork will be C4 "rock-step-kick-step-kick-step". Again, keep the kicks low, from the knee.

Starting from a closed, side-by-side position, take a rock step (1-2). Now both of you turn toward each other, "kick through" in-between each other's legs and step down on the kicking foot (3-4). You will kick with your LF outside her right leg and she will kick with her RF between your legs. On 5-6 repeat the "kick-through" with the other foot. This time you will kick between her legs while she kicks outside your right leg.

Now turn back side-to-side, do a rock step (1-2) and repeat the Jig Kicks, or do another figure.

You can also repeat the kick-throughs several times without a rock step. When you had enough, rock back on left foot to exit.

Keep the closed position closer than usual. For better effect, when you kick with your left foot you can dip your left hand a little, and when you kick with your right foot you can raise your left hand a little. You can also gradually rotate to right while doing the Jig Kicks, to add variety.

Lolly Kicks (or "Lollies")

Also known as Jig Walk, this figure has a simple footwork pattern: rock-step-kick-step-kick-step-kick-step.. for as long as you want.

Start from a side-by-side closed position with regular handhold. Lead a rock step (1-2) turning out a little. On 3, both of you turn toward each other, compress your hands and do a "kick through" (Jig kick). Step forward on 4. On 5, turn away from each other, stretch your handhold and kick away. Step forward on 6.

To avoid kicking each other on the cross-kicks, the lead should kick higher and outside the follower, while the follow should kick lower and through the lead's legs.

Keep walking forward in this fashion, kicking alternatingly in and out, towards and away from each other. The follower will mirror you so that you will be turning in and out at the same time.

You can also release your left hand, so that your only connection is your right arm around her waist, and lead the Lollies this way.

To exit, then step back on LF after a cross-kick to lead a rock-step.

Skip-Up (8c)

The Skip-Up is similar to the Lolly Kicks but it is more energetic, the kicks are progressively larger and when you kick with one foot, you jump forward on the other foot.

The kicks should gradually increase in strength and height. After the last cross-kick (7), do not step down, but rather keep your kicking left foot up in the air ("kick-hold").

This footwork pattern of the Skip-Up is: rock-step-kick-step-kick-step-kick-hold.

The Skip-Up is often followed by the Peel-Away.

Peel-Away (4c or 8c)

This is a natural way of exiting the Skip-Up.

After the last cross-kick (kick-gold with LF) of the Skip-Up, both of you will "peel" (turn) away from each other, using the momentum of the compressed hands, and do a 360 outside turn moving backwards in 4 counts (kick-step-kick-step, or simply:

step-hold-step-hold). This is a free turn for both of you, mirroring each other (left turn for you, right turn for her).

You initiate the follower's turn by a gentle pull with you right hand around her waist, not by pushing her away with your left hand.

At the end of your turns, you can either catch her hand when you reach a face-to-face open position, or turn a quarter more to end up side-by-side in closed position with your right arm around her waist. Either way, make sure to connect with her clearly, otherwise she may just continue turning.

You can also lead two full free turns instead of one, simply by not making contact after the first turn, in which case this will be a Double Peel-Away.

If you feel lazy, lead the follower into a Peel-Away but skip your own 360 left turn, turning instead a quarter to the right and taking a step to the right to catch her face-to-face when she is done with her turn ("Fake-Out Peel-Away").

The Peel-Away can also be added to other steps. If you simply add it to a rock-step-cross-kick, it can be used to change your position on the dance floor, or as a fun way to get from closed position into open position.

He-Goes-She-Goes (8c-C2 or C3)

This is the same step described previously under basic 8-count Lindy steps, but the triple-steps are replaced with kick-steps (C2 footwork).

If the figure is done with the Lindy Charleston footwork (C3), then the second rock step (5-6) is further replaced by kick-&.

Charleston Promenade (8c-C2 or C3)

This is the same as the Lindy Promenade but you replace the triple steps with kick steps (C2).

You can try the Charleston Promenade with Lindy Charleston (C3) footwork. In this case you will not progress much on the dance floor as you lose one "step" to a "kick".

Charleston Circle (8c-C2 or C3)

This is similar to the Lindy Circle but done with Charleston footwork.

Replace the triple steps with kick steps. The footwork is "rock-step-kick-step-rock-step-kick-step". The side-to-side position is a bit more separated than in the Lindy Circle to allow space for the kicks. Give a good stretch to the follower on 5-6, which is a rock step here (rather than a step-step in the Lindy Circle).

The Charleston Circle can also be done with the C3 Lindy Charleston footwork.

Charleston Tuck Turn (6c-C4 or 8c-C3)

These are the same as the 6-count or 8-count Lindy Tuck Turns but with the corresponding Charleston footwork.

When leading a 6-count Charleston Tuck Turn, bring down your left hand earlier to indicate that it is a 6-count move (just like with the regular Lindy Tuck Turn).

Charleston Change of Places (6c-C4 or 8c-C3)

The 6-count version is the same as the 6-count Lindy Change of Places but with the 6-count Charleston footwork: rock-step-kick-step-kick-step. Bring your left hand down before the second kick-step.

The 8-count version is the same as the 8-count Lindy Change of Places but with the 8-count Charleston footwork: rock-step-kick-step-kick-&-kick-step. Keep your left hand up until the last kick.

Charleston Side Pass (6c-C4)

This is the same as the 6-count hands-free Lindy Right Side Pass but with the 6-count Charleston footwork: rock-step-kick-step-kick-step. She will turn her back to you as she passes in front of you from left to right. Keep your kicks small.

The figure can be led both from a left-to-right or a right-to-right handshake handhold. In either case you will have to let go of her hand during the side pass, and then you are free to reconnect with the type of handhold that you need for your next move.

Charleston Cuddle (6c-C4 or 8c-C2)

The 6-count version is the same as the 6-count Lindy Cuddle but with the 6-count Charleston footwork: rock-step-kick-step-kick-step.

The 8-count version is the same as the 8-count Lindy Cuddle but with the 8-count Charleston footwork: rock-step-kick-step-rock-step-kick-step.

Footwork variations

Footwork variations are easy and fun to learn and make a big difference both in the enjoyment and the appearance of your dance. They are really the spice and seasoning of the dance that can give a unique flavour and character to an otherwise bland figure.

They are slight variations of your footwork within the existing structure of a figure and do not change the structure of the figure. There is not a lot to explain about footwork variations, you just have to practice them until they are committed to muscle memory.

The only important thing you need to be conscious of is the type of the step you want to replace with a footwork variation, namely whether it is a straight step or a change step. As explained before, straight steps involve an even number of weight changes (typically 0 or 2), while change steps involve an odd number of weight changes (typically 1 or 3). The rhythm pattern of the replacement footwork does not matter, but the number of weight changes does.

As long as the footwork variations conform to the type of the steps they replace or modify, they should not affect the timing of the steps.

If two or more footwork variations follow each other, you need to make sure that you have the desired number of weight changes in total, i.e. an even number or an odd number. For example "step-step-triple-step" can be replaced by a single step or a slide.

You can also transform the same footwork variation from a change step to a straight step (and vice versa) by tacking on another weight change, usually at the end.

Footwork variations should not affect your lead, i.e. they should not change what the follower feels.

Footwork variations can be applied by one partner independently or by both partners simultaneously. It can look great if applied by both partners at the same time, but since they are not "led" this is difficult to pull off unless you are dancing with someone who knows your dance habits.

Footwork variations can be applied to almost any standard Lindy move and they can be done practically anywhere within a figure. The easiest places to vary the footwork are those where the dancer is stationary or does not travel much, such as in the rock step.

STRAIGHT STEP VARIATIONS

These variations have an even number of weight changes, and you end up with your weight on the same foot where you started from.

Stomp Off

The Stomp Off usually marks the end of a pause or some kind of slow-down in the dance. It is done on "&8". With your weight on your right foot, jump in place very slightly. Your left foot will hit the ground first (&), and your right foot second (8), slightly behind the left foot. The move gives you a backward momentum in preparation for a rock step.

You can use the Stomp Off while pulsing in closed position with your follower to signal to her the lead-in beat in preparation for the start of a dance.

You can also close off a slide that lasts a couple of beats, with a Stomp Off to signal the end of the slide and the beginning of the next step.

Hold

This means that you simply miss a rock step or step-step (usually 1-2 or 5-6), maintaining your weight on one foot instead.

Kick-And

This is a variation to the rock step in open position, without a weigh change. Very effective as the start of a Swingout.

Maintain your weight on your right foot. On 1, lean slightly back right (giving your partner a good stretch), kick forward left with your left foot, and raise your right hand reaching up. On 2, lift your left knee slightly, preparing to launch forward on the next triple-step.

This variation works best when it follows some other footwork variation on 7&8. It is also useful when there is not enough space behind you for a rock step.

You can also kick sideway to left, or turn to the right and kick toward right ("Kick-Away"), as your dancing and styling calls for it.

The Bow

This too is a variation on the rock step in open position, without a weigh change. On 1, with your left foot slightly in front, straighten your legs, take a deep bow and swing your right arm back. Re-compose and flex your knees on 2.

Heel Pops (or just "Heels")

The Heel Pops is a version of the Bow. It too replaces the rock step and is done in open, face-to-face position. Have your feet side by side. On 1, lift your toes and stay on both heels, lean slightly forward, stick out your butt and swing your right arm back. On 2, drop your toes and get back on your feet, swing your right arm forward and prepare for the triple step.

The Heel Pops can also replace a step-step, as for example in the 8-count Sugar Push.

Jump Stop (4c)

This is a "jump and freeze" that brings a figure to a quick halt. It is a good way to mark a break in the song or to prepare for jazz steps.

In a side-by-side closed position, do a rock step (1-2). On 3, both of you step forward, turn somewhat toward each other, bend your knees and lower your level. On 4, both of you take a small jump away from each other. On 5-8, you can either freeze or do break steps.

The Jump Stop can replace the second part of the Swingout. Lower your level on 5 and jump back (away from each other) on 6. Hold on 7-8. Continue with jazz steps.

Slide Out

The Slide Out also brings a figure to a quick halt. Start in a face-to-face closed position.

On 1, take a small jump landing on both legs with bent knees. On 2, slide both feet out to side, keeping your head level.

This can be done at the end of many figures, for example at 7-8 of the Swingout. If done on 5-6 of a figure, just freeze on 7-8.

Step-Overs

Replace the rock step, for example at the beginning of a Swingout, with two cross-steps.

Start in open position. On 1, step with your left foot in front and across your right foot, turning right. On 2, turn left and step with your right foot in front and across your left foot. On 3, continue with a triple step.

Kick-Ball-Change

The Kick-Ball-Change (1&2) replaces a rock step or step-step. It consists of a kick (1) followed by a "ball-change" (&2). It can start on either foot, depending on the step that is being varied.

Kick with your free foot on 1. Keep the kick low, from the knee, not from the hip.

"Ball" (&) means that after the kick you jump up slightly from the supporting foot and land on the ball of your kicking foot, often placing it behind the jumping foot. "Change" (2) means that you step down and slightly ahead with the original supporting foot. You end with your weight on the original supporting foot.

The "Ball" will carry very little of your body weight as it is followed immediately by the "Change" where your full body weigh lands.

Assuming you start with your weight on your RF, you will kick with LF (1), jump from RF and land on the ball of LF with little weight (&), then immediately land on RF with full weight (2).

Ball-Change

The Ball-Change is a Kick-Ball-Change without the kick. Instead of kicking, just hold (i.e. don't do anything) on 1, and do the Ball-Change on "&2".

This is similar to the Stomp Off but the "Ball" lands somewhat behind your supporting foot.

Double Ball-Change

Instead of kicking or holding on 1, you can do a Ball-Change on 1 as well. Now you will have two quick Ball-Changes (&1&2).

CHANGE STEP VARIATIONS

These footwork variations end with your weight on the other foot than where you started from.

Hold-Step or Step-Hold

You can replace a triple-step with just one single step. You can step on either the first or the second beat, and hold on the other. Don't forget to pulse.

Eagle Slide

Step forward on one foot (1), then jump and slide forward on the same foot with knee bent and arms raised and spread like the wings of an eagle landing (2). Add an eagle cry for better effect.

Kick-Step

This footwork variation can be used, for example, to replace the "7&8" triple step of the Swingout. Instead of the triple step, kick to the side and slightly forward on 7 with your right foot, leaning back slightly. Then step back on your right foot on 8.

The Sweep

Also called "Leg Sweep" or "Ronde". This can also be a variation for the closing "7&8" of a Swingout. Instead of the triple step, draw (sweep) a semi-circle with your right toes on your right side, maintaining your weight on your left foot. The semi-circle will start in front of your left foot and end behind it. Transfer your weight to your right foot at the end of the Sweep.

From here, you can continue with a rock step (1-2), or replace it with another footwork variation. This could be a Kick, or you could do another Sweep with your left foot, this time maintaining your weight on your right foot.

The Sweep can be a straight step variation if you maintain your weight on one foot and do not transfer it to the other foot at the end of the Sweep.

Side Slide

With your full weight on one leg, flex that leg and drop your weight a little. Push off from that foot sideways into the opposite direction, sliding on the free foot and raising the leading shoulder. Transfer your weight to the sliding foot and get into upright position, drawing in the pushing leg.

This step can be used as a variation during the second half of an 8-count figure, and it is also suitable for ending a dance. Push off on 5 and slide on 6-7-8.

COMBINED STEP VARIATIONS

Scissor Kicks

This consists of two continuous "sideway" Kick-Ball-Changes on 7&8 (to right) and 1-2 (to left). It is often used to connect two Swingouts. You end one Swingout with a Kick-Ball-Change on 7&8, and start the next one with another Kick-Ball-Change on 1&2.

Kick first with your RF, to your right, on 7. This comes fairly early in the first Swingout, so be prepared for it. The "Change" will be in front and across your RF, moving right.

Since a Kick-Ball-Change is a straight-step footwork variation, you will have to add one quick step-down on RF (&) in order to switch legs, before the second Kick-Ball-Change.

On 1, start the second Kick-Ball-Change by kicking with your LF slightly to the left. The "Change" will be in front and across your LF, moving left. After the Kick-Ball-Change, continue with the usual 3&4 triple-step forward.

Your 7&8&1&2 pattern will then be: "Kick-Ball-Change-&-Kick-Ball-Change".

The Scissor Kicks look great if you can do them together with your follower, mirroring each other, giving each other a good stretch.

Kick-Step & Kick-Away

Do a Kick-Step on 7&8 of a Swingout and a Kick-Away on 1-2 of the next Swingout.

The Snap

This is another great way to connect two Swingouts.

On "7" of a Swingout, take a single step on your RF. On "8", lift your left knee and snap the fingers of your right hand turning to the right and giving your follower a stretch.

Hold on "1", do a Ball-Change on "&2", and continue with the usual triple step on "3&4".

Break or jazz steps

During a dance you or your partner may decide to temporarily separate by releasing physical contact entirely. During these short "breaks", both dancers have the freedom to dance independently and do their own thing. The steps or short step combinations one commonly performs during these breaks are called "break steps". They are also called "jazz steps" or "solo jazz steps".

Separating from and then reuniting with your follower adds variety to the dance. Separation ideally occurs as a result of a conscious decision on part of the lead (or sometimes on part of the follower). Good places to separate are the ones where a figure requires you to release contact anyway, such as a Belt Turn. Just don't grab her hand after the turn is completed, and you are separated.

Reconnecting with your partner is done either by taking her hand in an open, face-to-face position, or getting on her left side and putting your right arm around her waist to get into closed position, typically in preparation of a rock step.

It is not necessary to completely separate in order to do break steps. You can also do them when you are in a loose open position (such as at the end of a Swingout). You can then decide to maintain that position instead of bringing her in for another step, or it may be that the follower decides on her own to "take a break" in this fashion. This gives you enough freedom to do your own thing while keeping a loose hand-to-hand connection.

Many break steps can be led very effectively using a double handhold as it enables strong compression and stretch with the follower. Side-to-side is also a good position for many break steps as it provides close contact for an effective lead.

Often, separation occurs as a result of a mistake, a small misunderstanding, indecisive lead or ineffective following. If this happens, there is no reason to panic. It is better to roll with the punches and treat it as an opportunity to do some break steps until you re-connect.

There is a great variety of popular break or jazz steps. Many of them come from tap dancing. Some are short and simple, well suited for the temporary breaks in the dance, while others are more complex and better suited for choreographed routines.

Many break steps traditionally start on beat 8 (the last beat of the previous figure).

Some break steps are stationary, done in one place, on a spot; others cover a small distance forward, backward or sideways. You can regulate the length of travel by the size of your steps. Choosing very small steps, even travelling jazz steps can be done almost in place. Steps moving backward and steps moving forward can be linked naturally.

Although the most popular break steps can be learned, break steps in general are an opportunity for self-expression. It is good to know some so that you have tools to choose from, but the best jazz steps are what the music drives one to do, and everyone is welcome to make up their own.

The break steps listed below are short and simple enough to be useful in social dancing. First come a few steps that are done in place, and then a few more that involve moving around (the direction is noted in brackets after the name of the step). Both types are useful depending on the situation.

66

Mess Around

Stand with feet slightly apart, knees flexed. Put your hands on your hips and rock your hips around in a circle, bouncing down once per beat and completing the circle on 8. You can do this clockwise or counter clockwise.

Step Tap

Step Taps are very easy, and they serve well as "go-to" steps when you find yourself in a situation that calls for break steps – and nothing comes to mind.

On 1, step to left on LF, keeping your leg straight. On 2, close your right foot to the left without weight and tap on the floor, bending your left knee. Do not step down. Now step to right on RF and do the mirror image (3-4). Repeat as desired. The footwork is "step-tap-step-tap". Remember to pulse (dip) on each tap.

This can be done facing your follower in an open position, in which case you will mirror each other. You can also stand shoulder-to-shoulder (left-to-left or right-to-right), in which case you will step and tap towards and away from each other.

Heel Tap

Heel Taps are also easy to do and are great "go-to" steps.

Stand with feet slightly apart. On 1, tap forward on the floor with your left heel, turning your toes out to left. On 2, step to the side on LF. On 3, tap forward on the floor with your right heel, turning your toes to right. On 4, step to the side on your RF. Repeat as desired.

You can also tap diagonally across and in front of your supporting foot, then step down in your original position (instead of stepping to the side).

The footwork is "tap-step-tap-step". Keep pulsing and dip on every "tap".

Tacky Annie

This is the opposite of the Heel Tap. Instead of tapping forward with your heel, tap the floor behind you with your toes. Bend your supporting knee on every tap. The footwork is again "tap-step-tap-step".

Lift your elbows to the side, forearms pointing forward, and move your elbows backwards on each tap, like you are pulling something towards you on every tap.

You can also do your toe taps across and behind the supporting leg.

Lowdown

On 1, small jump in place landing on left foot with a bent knee, and sliding out your right foot to the side. Hold on 2. On 3, small jump in place landing on right foot with bent knee and sliding out your left foot to the side. Hold on 4. Repeat as desired.

Boogie Drops

Tap the floor with the ball of your left foot twice to your left, gradually turning your body to left (1-2), then on the third tap drop your weight, bending both knees, facing left (3). Hold on 4. Turn to right and repeat on the other side.

As you turn your upper body toward the tapping side, push out your hip into that direction and make each tap a little further away from you.

Alternatively, do a toe tap in place (1), do a heel tap turning left (2), then step out to left and drop your weight with knees bent. Repeat on the other side.

Cross-Overs

Do a rock step on 1-2. Kick forward with your left foot on 3, and step down diagonally across, in front of your right foot on 4. Repeat on the other side.

This can be done while separated, or in open position facing your partner. Do it in a double handhold, so that you can compress against your partner on 3.

You can also do this move side-by-side, leading it with your right arm around her waist. Move alternatingly toward and away from each other. Exit into another figure after a left foot rock step, or step forward after a right foot rock step and freeze.

Applejacks

Keep marching in place with strong pulsing. Step down on the ball of your foot on each beat at an even pace, with toes pointing inward. After each step-down, swivel on your heel, turning your toes outward.

This results in a twisting body motion like you are trying to put out a cigarette butt or push something into the ground. Exaggerate the movement of the hips and knees, and swing your arms naturally as the twists require.

Jazz Box

The rhythm of this figure is an even 1-2-3-4.

Step with left foot across and in front of right foot (1). Step back on RF (2), then step to the side on LF (3), and finally step forward on RF (4), completing the box. Bend your knee and lean forward on the step-back (beat 2). Exaggerate the swinging of your arms.

You can also do the Jazz Box the other way around, starting with right foot stepping across in front of the left foot.

Lock Turn

Stand with feet slightly apart, weight split evenly. Jump in place, turning your lower body a quarter to left in the air, and lend with knees bent (squat), right leg crossed in front of left. Your torso and face is still facing the original direction.

Transfer you weight to your left (back) foot and unwind yourself by pivoting a full turn to left until you once again face your original direction. Close your right foot to the left foot during the pivot.

This is easier said than done as it requires good body isolation, and you will need some practice to get it right without losing your balance.

The Lock Turn can also be done rotating to right.

Tick Tocks

These are toe taps while swiveling on your heels.

Stand with feet slightly apart, weight on your heels. Keep tapping on the floor with the toes of both feet, at an even beat, at the same time, but in different directions. Tap first with toes pointing inward (pigeon toes), then with toes pointing out. Keep swiveling on your heels to accommodate the taps. Repeat as desired: toes together-apart-together-apart. You will stay on the same spot while doing this.

You can also do the Tick Tocks moving sideways. This is a bit trickier. The toes will still move "together-apart-together-apart" but this time one foot will swivel on the heel and the other foot on the ball, changing alternatingly.

Truckin' (forward)

This step comes from an old swing dance called "Truckin" (or "Truckin' on Down").

Truckin' moves you forward on the dance floor at an even pace, in a rhythmic zig-zag pattern, turning alternatingly slightly right and slightly left.

Step with left foot in front of the right, turning your body 1/8 to right (1). Swivel on your left heel a quarter to the left (2). Step forward on right foot (3). Swivel on your right heel a quarter to right (4). Repeat as desired.

Put your left hand on your stomach or on your hip, and point up with your right index finger. Wag that index finger while you do the Truckin'.

Boxy Suit (forward)

Stand with your arms to your side, index fingers pointing down, shoulders raised.

Step with your left foot in front of the right and lean your upper body to left to keep it in line with the stepping leg (pretending that you have a stiff body). Now step with the right foot across the left and lean your upper body to right.

Keep doing this as long as desired and change the direction of your travel as it suits your dancing or the space on the dance floor. You can step on every beat for a faster walk or on every second beat for a slower walk.

Shorty George (forward)

I mention this as it is a popular break step but I would not recommend it because it is too hard on the knees if not done properly.

Knee Slaps (forward)

Walk forward at an even pace, lifting your knee at every step and slapping it with your hand. Slap left knee with left hand, right knee with right hand.

Skating (forward)

This involves small repeated jumps on the same foot in a zig-zag pattern. It mimics the long strides of ice skating.

Step down forcefully on your left foot, forward and 45° to the left, and do three small jumps on the same foot into that same direction (quick-quick-quick-quick), left hand pointing to the direction of your jumps, right hand on your hip.

Repeat stepping down on right foot, a quarter to the right, your right hand pointing, left hand on your hip.

Boogie Forward (forward)

Kick forward with LF on 8 (the closing beat of the preceding figure), roll your hip in a semi-circle forward and to left and step forward on 1. Kick forward with RF on 2, bring your hip around and step forward on 3. Continue forward in this fashion on 4-5 and 6-7.

On each step, emphasize the circular hip motion by pushing it out forward and rolling it to the side of your stepping leg.

For better effect, roll back your shoulders on each kick, or push out your elbows to the side and let your forearms dangle.

The natural continuation of the Boogie Forward is the Boogie Back.

Boogie Back (backward)

Bend your knees and squat down just a little.

Clap on 8 (the closing beat of the preceding figure) and shuffle back on "&1". The shuffle consists of a small jump back lending on left foot and closing the right foot. Keep repeating: clap-shuffle (&2), clap-shuffle (&3) and so on.

If you add a small kick at the same time when you clap, then this becomes a series of Kick-Ball-Changes travelling backward.

Fishtail (backward)

This is a simple and useful break step that takes you backwards in a zig-zag pattern.

Stand with feet slightly apart.

On 1, step back and out to the side on your left foot and flex your left knee. On 2, swivel a bit to the left on your left heel while straightening you left leg and closing your right foot to the left. On 3, step back on your right foot and flex your knee. On 4, swivel a bit to the right on your right heel while straightening you right leg and closing your left foot to the right. Repeat.

Keep your upper body facing forward throughout. Move your arms naturally, and you can clap on every swivel (2, 4, etc) if you wish.

Fall off the Log (sideways)

This step starts on the last beat (usually beat 8) of the preceding figure.

Kick to the right with your RF on 8, turning your body right and leaning slightly back. This looks like you are losing your balance and falling back, hence the name. On 1, step back on RF crossing behind LF. On 2, step to left on your LF. On 3, step to left with your RF in crossing in front of LF.

Now do this from left to right, starting with a kick to the left with your left foot on 4. The footwork pattern is "kick-cross-step-cross" x 2. Clap on every kick.

To exit, wait for beat 7 when your weight is on your left foot. On beat 8, instead of kicking to the side, step down on your right foot, and you are ready for the next figure.

Suzy Q (sideways)

Also spelled Susie Q or Suzie Q, this step originated from a novelty dance of the same name.

- Start on beat 8 with a small kick with RF out to the right
- On 1, step to left on RF, toes pointing left, crossing in front of LF with flexed knees
- On 2, step left on LF crossing behind RF and swivel your RF to turn toes to right
- Repeat the side steps, travelling to left (3-4-5-6-7)

On 8, kick with your left foot out to left and do a mirror image of the above procedure, this time travelling sideways to right.

With the exception of the side-kicks, keep your knees bent. Clap your hands on each step on back foot. The front foot swivels left and right at each step. The back foot takes simple steps to the side without swiveling.

As a variation, hold your foot in the air after the side kick for two beats and step down only on 3. From here, move sideways as usual.

The Suzy Q can be led in various positions. Side-by-side with your partner is very effective. So is facing each other in closed position and doing the Suzy Q in a small circle.

Side Crawl (sideways)

In this figure, you will slowly crawl to left with your weight on you left foot, then crawl to right with your weight on you right foot.

Stand with feet slightly apart.

On 1, step to the left with heel leading (toes pointing right or inward). Step down firmly, with your weight on your left heel and bend your left knee. Keep your right leg straight, toes pointing to right and touching the floor without weight.

On 2, swivel on your left heel, turn your left toes outward and shift your weight to the ball of your left foot. Keep your upper body facing forward and your right leg straight.

On 3, swivel on the ball of your left foot (turning toes inward again) and shift your weight to your left heel. This will move (crawl) you slightly to the left. Keep your upper body facing forward and your right leg straight.

Repeat this swiveling and weight shifting between heel and ball at an even pace (4-5-6-7-8), crawling sideways to left, dragging your straight right leg after you.

Now repeat the same, this time crawling to right with your weight on your bent right leg and dragging your straight left leg after you.

Let your arms move naturally at your side, as if you were running.

Repetitive steps

I use the term "repetitive steps" to refer to any part of a dance figure repeated several times.

The point of using repetitive steps is to add surprise and variety to the dance. Like any ingredient of a good composition, it has its place and its good measure in the dance, so use them when they go well with the music, but do not overdo them.

In addition to bringing variety to the dance, these steps are also useful when the music is fast and you want to "take a break" from the hectic action.

Keep pulsing during repetitive steps just like during regular figures.

Checked movements

A "checked movement" means that a figure is stopped (checked) at one point, and a part of it is reversed and then repeated one or more times before the figure is then continued and completed.

A checked movement interrupts a normal figure to "re-play" just a small portion of it.

Many Lindy figures can be checked, so keep an open mind and look for opportunities.

As an example, on 5-6 in a Swingout, instead of stepping out of the follower's way, you can step back to check her (5) and hold for one beat (6), then step forward to lead her back to her previous position (7) and hold for one beat there (8), before continuing with the regular 5-8 counts (which will now be 9-12).

You can repeat the checked part more than once, which will extend the original figure even further.

Freeze

The Freeze is a deliberate stopping of a step or sequence. For example, do a rock-step, then step down firmly on 3 and freeze the motion until the end of an 8-count phrase.

"Freezing" does not mean that movement stops completely. While you do not perform any particular step, you should continue pulsing to the music.

A Freeze is also a useful aid when you get mixed up with your steps and need a short break and a clean start to sort them out.

Continuous Lindy Circle

This is a regular Lindy Circle, but you keep repeating the "step-step" of 5-6 a couple of times before doing the final triple step.

Keep up the rotation of the Lindy Circle during the additional steps.

Kick-Back

This is a simple figure that can be used to mark the end of a musical phrase, to break the monotony of rotating steps, or to get back into rhythm after a mistake.

Start from side-by-side closed position. Kick forward with your left foot, then step down. Kick back with your right foot, then step down. Repeat. The rhythm is even 8 counts: 2 x "kick-step-kick-step".

Lean slightly back when you kick forward and lean slightly forward when you kick back. Keep your kicks low and hold your follower firmly throughout. Make sure nobody is behind you when you kick back.

Cat Walk

Start from side-by-side closed position, without holding hands. Lead a rock step, then step forward and across on left foot turning slightly toward the follower, leading her to mirror you and turn toward you. Then step forward and across on right foot turning away from her, leading her to do the same. Keep marching forward in single steps, hitting each beat in this fashion.

You will lead this figure only with your right hand around her waist and with the twisting of your body right and left. Your left hand remaining free throughout.

To exit, wait for the next cross-step on LF and replace it with a triple-step turning right and moving in front of the follower. Take her hand, and you are now ready to step back on RF and lead the second half of a Swingout.

Add another triple step while turning further right, and you are now back in normal open position, ready for a rock step on LF.

Pimp Walk

You can do the Pimp Walk alone, or walking together with your partner in a closed, side-by-side position.

To walk together, start in an open position with right-to-right "handshake" handhold. Do a rock step (1-2) and lead a Right Side Pass (3&4), keeping your hand low and holding on to her hand as she does her turn. This will roll her to your side in a 'sweetheart" position. On 5, start walking forward, stepping on every second beat (5&-7&-1&-3&..). Dip a little on every step, angle your upper body slightly to right, lean slightly forward and put your left hand behind your back.

If you walk alone, the Pimp Walk serves as a break step. Let your right hand swing freely and snap with your fingers on every step. Give it some attitude.

Washing Machine

Start in an open position with R2R cross handhold, and do a rock step.

On 1 of the rock step, turn a quarter to your left and extend your right hand forward, leading the follower into a rock step with a quarter turn of her own. This winds up both of you for the next step.

On 3&4, triple-step almost in place, turn your body a quarter to right and pull in your right hand, down and to your right in a semi-circle. At the same time raise your left hand and tap her back as she triples forward making a quarter turn away from you and showing you her back.

On 5&6, triple-step almost in place, turning a quarter to left and swinging your right hand down and to your left. This will make her turn towards you while she triples, and she may now tap on your back. At this point your left hand is free.

Repeat the triple-steps, still holding hands R2R, turning alternatingly towards and away from each other like the agitator of a washing machine, moving slowly in a clockwise circle around the axis between you.

To exit, use the next triple-step turning towards her to lead a free Right Side Pass. Let go of her hand so that she can do a free turn. While she turns, do another triple step to your right and catch her hand at the end of her turn.

You can do a full right turn of your own during this second triple step if you wish.

Switches

The Switches is a popular figure and typically follows an overturned Swingout, but it can be led from any overturned open position. During this figure, you stay at the centre and the follower moves around you in a wide circle like a carousel.

Do a Swingout. On 8, turn the follower out to her left by extending your left hand diagonally and turning your palm down. From here, lead her in a circle around you in clockwise direction, keeping a good stretch throughout, while she is swiveling (twisting) continuously as she progresses around you. You lead the swivels by alternatingly turning your left hand palm-up and palm-down (as if turning a key). Your arm will not move much, only your hand.

You can choose your own footwork while leading the Switches. To keep it simple, take small, rocking single steps in-place, left foot behind the right, while slowly rotating to your right. Or you can tap back with alternating feet (as if doing a Tacky Annie while rotating in-place). Keep your knees bent throughout.

Lead the Switches for 8 or 16 beats. 8 beats will cover roughly one full circle.

Chicken Walks

This step is borrowed from Jive and East Coast Swing. It starts similar to the Switches but this time you will pull the follower toward you as you back away, rather than in a circle around you.

Lead the follower into an overturned open position. This can be a simple overturned 6-count Sendout where on 5&6 you extend your left hand diagonally and turn your palm down. This will prompt her to turn out to her left.

Now take six steps backwards. The rhythm is "slow-slow-quick-quick-quick-quick". On every step, swivel your wrist slightly left and right (as if turning a key). She will follow you as you back away, swiveling, twisting her hips left and right, pointing her toes out on every step and doing styling with her free hand (or putting it on her hip). During your back steps, apply some "Merengue-style" hip action.

To exit, just pull her up on her last step and do a rock step to start a next figure. Or continue into two triple-steps leading her into an underarm turn passing in front of you left to right (the 3&4-5&6 of the 6-count Change of Places).

Neither the number of steps nor the rhythm pattern are cast in stone. You can vary them as you feel it suits the music.

Make sure not to back into anyone on the dance floor. If there is not enough space behind you, the step can still be done. Instead of backing away, you stay more or less in one place and lead a pulling-and-pushing. She will do her steps and swivels sideways, also staying in one place.

Paddle

This figure has no triple-steps. Instead, you both will be rotating counter-clockwise in a small circle, facing each other and using your left foot as your common axis.

Start in side-by-side closed position, and do a rock step (1-2).

On 3, step forward forcefully on left foot, lean forward and to your left and bring your left hand down sharply, leading the follower to step in front of you and turn to face you. This movement stops the follower from doing a triple step. Hold one beat in this position (4).

On 5, rise on the ball of your right foot, and start moving (one step per beat) in a small circle counter-clockwise. Keep your LF on one spot flat on the floor, and "paddle" around it by going up on the ball of your RF, and down flat on your LF (anchor foot). Up on RF (5), down on LF (6) and so on.

The follower, facing you, will mirror what you do. She will paddle around her right foot which is placed close to your left foot, forming a common axis. She will step back on LF when you step forward on RF.

While doing this, swing your left forearm back-and-forth as if paddling, keeping it parallel to the floor, extending your arm forward when you rise on RF and pulling it back when you lower onto LF. Since you do this with her hand in yours, you will be paddling together. She should keep her arm relaxed and offer no resistance, to avoid discomfort or injury. As you paddle, look to the left, towards the centre of the circle.

This is a repetitive step because you can paddle in this fashion, at an even pace, up-down-up-down, for as long as you like.

To exit the Paddle, release your right hand from the follower's back, turn gradually right to face her, and let her separate while still holding hands. Give her a good stretch and bring her in for a Lindy Circle.

Kick-Through Charleston (C3)

Also known as "Charleston Kick-Aways". Do a side-by-side Charleston Basic. On 5 (forward kick with your right foot), move your right hand from your partner's waist to her inside hip. Push it slightly away from you on "&" and pivot 180° to your right on 6-

7. She will mirror you and pivot 180° to her left. Step down on 8 in this new direction.

From here, the footwork changes to "kick-&-kick-step" in a repeat fashion, while doing half-turns left and right. You always kick forward, but after each "kick" with your inside leg, you will pivot 180° left or right, turning towards your partner ("&"), and finish the "kick-step" in the new direction. She will mirror you throughout.

Keep holding her right hand with your left hand. After each pivot to left, put your right hand back on her hip to push on it again to facilitate the next pivot to right.

There are many ways to exit the Kick-Through. On a pivot to left, instead of putting your hand on her hip, you can slide your arm around her waist and ease back into side-by-side Charleston Basic.

Another way to exit on a pivot to left, is to raise your left hand and lead her into an underarm turn. You can add an underarm turn of your own if your wish. Make sure your footwork falls in place at the end and your left foot is free for the next move, so your finishing footwork may be something like kick-step-kick-hold.

Switching your footwork is an issue with many Charleston steps and getting it right requires some practice and experience.

Kick-Through with Turns (C3)

Turns can be added to the Kick-Through Charleston for variety or to facilitate an exit. The turns can be to the right or to the left. You will start the turns when you step down after a pivot.

Whether the pivot is to the left or to the right, don't stop the turning momentum. Let go of her hand and do a free turn travelling slightly downline in the direction of the pivot. A full turn will take 4 beats and the footwork is kick-step-kick-step. She will mirror you, doing a turn with the same footwork. Catch her hand again at the end of the turn, or continue with another turn if there is enough room on the dance floor.

At the end of each turn you have the opportunity to catch her hand and either go back to doing Kick-Throughs or exiting by doing some other step. For example, after doing a right turn, you can ease into a side-by-side Charleston Basic.

You can do turns alternatingly left and right. At the end of a turn, catch her hand and swing her back in the opposite direction.

You can also lead her into a turn after pivoting to right without following her. Instead, do a kick-step-kick-step in place and catch her left hand at the end of her turn. You are now in a face-to-face open position and out of the Kick-Through, ready to do a rock step, for example.

Pancake Charleston (C3)

Also referred to as "Hand-to-Hand Charleston", this is a further variant of the Kick-Through. This time, you and your partner will kick into opposite directions with the same foot. You can think of it as reverse Kick-Throughs.

Get into the "pancake" position by skipping one of your pivots during the Charleston Kick-Through while letting your partner do hers. You just keep kicking (2 additional "kick-&") while she pivots, then you resume your normal steps and pivots. You are now kicking into opposite directions which also changes the handhold from normal to cross-handhold (alternating R2R and L2L). Your hands meet temporarily, palm to palm and compress against each other, helping your pivots.

Do not stay too close to each other and remember to pulse. Your two additional kicks on the switch to Pancake may be both forward, or one back and one forward.

As always, there are many ways to get out of the Hand-to-Hand Charleston. You can simply exit the way you entered, by skipping a pivot and reverting to Kick-Throughs.

Another way to exit is to do a "Butterfly". When you get to the next R2R handhold, swing your right foot forward and your right hand back-and-up to signal the end of the move (1-2), then use that momentum to do a right-foot rock step for a good stretch (3-4). From here, lead the follower into a hands-free Charleston Side Pass on 5-6-7-8 while you keep facing the same direction. Your footwork on 5-6-7-8 will be "kick-step-kick-&". When she turns side-by-side with you, catch her with your right arm around her waist, do a rock step, and you are back to side-by-side Charleston Basic.

Airplane Charleston (C3)

This figure (also known as Swoop) is somewhat similar to the Kick-Through Charleston but the footwork and the handhold are different.

It starts similar to the Kick-Through Charleston: Do a Charleston Basic side-by side. On 5 (forward kick with your right foot), move your right hand from your partner's waist to her inside hip. Push it slightly away from you on "&" and pivot 180° to your right on 6-7. She will mirror you and pivot 180° to her left. Step down on 8 in this new direction.

From here, the footwork changes to "kick-step-kick-&" (versus "kick-&-kick-step" in the Kick-Through) for as long as you wish. You will always kick forward, but after each kick with your outside leg, you will pivot 180° towards your partner and finish the "kick-

&" in the new direction. After the pivots to left do not put your right hand on her hip. Maintain an open position, switching between L2R and R2L handholds. You can also keep double handhold throughout the figure. Stay slightly further away from your partner than in the Kick-Through.

You can enter the Airplane Charleston in other ways, for example from a Charleston Tuck Turn. Turn to right on the second "kick-step" and get side-by-side with your follower, facing the same direction.

To get out of the Airplane Charleston, wait for a pivot to your left. After the pivot, instead of stepping forward, put your right arm around her waist and resume 4-8 of the Charleston Basic to ease back into side-by-side Charleston Basic.

Alternatively, after a pivot to left, pull back your right hand, check her and lead her into a spin counter-clockwise while holding her hand. This will roll her into your right arm and you can now walk together. Add some style by doing a "Pimp Walk".

Try switching between Kick-Throughs and Pancake Charleston by changing the footwork after a pivot.

Drunken Charleston

This is done in a side-by-side closed position. You will start with a Charleston Basic and switch to sideway crossovers to left and right.

Do a Charleston Basic. In preparation for the Drunken Charleston, align your steps with your follower's by switching from your own Charleston Basic footwork to hers. This is done on beat 7 by replacing kick-&-kick-step with kick-&-step-step (one extra weight change). This will allow both of you to move in the same sideway direction.

Once you switched legs, continue the Charleston Basic with a right-foot rock step. On 4, cross your right foot over your left foot and "fall" to the left, leading the follower to do the same and "dragging" her with you. Rock back from LF and repeat the cross-over to the opposite direction (to right). You can repeat the "Drunken Charleston" a couple of times. Your footwork will be "rock-step-kick-cross".

To exit the Drunken Charleston, get back into Charleston Basic and switch back to your regular footwork using the same switching procedure described above.

It is possible to do the Drunken Charleston with you regular footwork, without switching legs. Your sideway movements will now be falling away from each other and then falling towards each other, which can also be fun. Finish this version by stepping forward and dropping your knee on 7 and then freezing on 8 (this is called "Johnny's Drop").

Bonus Lindy figures

This chapter includes additional Lindy figures that you can use to make your dancing richer and more varied. The counts for each figure are given in brackets.

Side Chassés (8c)

This is often done on the second half of a Lindy Circle.

Do the first half of the Lindy Circle (1 to 4). By 4, face your partner, release your right hand and raise it slightly to the side (which gives a visual cue of the direction of the coming move).

From here, chassé to the right on the next 4 counts (5-&6-&7-&8). The follower will raise her left hand and chassé to her left, mirroring you.

As you chassé along, look at your right hand pointing the way, raise it gradually higher, and gradually move away from the follower to end the figure in an open position and to set up a stretch for the start of the next step.

This figure can be varied by replacing the chassé with a compatible footwork variation as you move along to your right. For example, you can do a "Kick-Ball-Change & Side Slide" instead of the chassés. Kick to the side (5), do a Ball-Change stepping with your left foot across and in front of your right foot (&6), then bend your left knee and push yourself into a long slide to the right to finish the move (7-8).

Swingback (8c)

This figure starts just like a Swingout, but this time the two of you will not swing around each other. Instead, you will check (stop) the follower's movement as she is about to pass you, and send her back the way she came.

Lead the first half of a Swingout from open position (1-4), but on 4 do not make a half turn to face the follower. Instead, only do a quarter turn to right and catch her back with your extended right hand just as she turned and passed by you. Your weight is on your flexed left leg to counter-balance the check and to give her a stretch.

On 5, swing her back, in front of you to the left, along the same path where she came from. She will turn 180 to left as she returns to her original position, and you will turn a quarter to left to face her again at the end. Both of you will end up on the same spot where you started from.

Swing-Not (8c)

This figure also starts like a Swingout from open position, except this time you will abandon the Swingout halfway through. You can surprise the follower with this move.

Lead the first half of a Swingout from open position (1-4). On 4, turn to face her and check her movement as usual, but then simply let go of her back, leave her there and back away into open position without swinging her out (5-6-7&8). She should stay where you left her or back away slightly.

This figure covers a half turn instead of a full turn for both of you, and you will trade places compared to your starting positions.

Fakeout (8c)

This is a "fake Swingout", another abandoned Swingout, but here you won't even touch the follower with your right hand.

Start from open position and pretend that you are going to lead a Swingout. Extend you right hand as if preparing to catch her on 4, but then just let her slide by without touching her. She should continue on her path, effectively trading places with you.

Lasso (8c or 6c)

The Lasso starts similar to the Swingout but this time you will lead the follower in a circle around you while you keep facing your original direction without turning.

Lead the first half of a Swingout from open position (1-4), but do not turn on 3&4. Instead, raise your left hand up across your chest and over your head in a wide circle (like swinging a lasso with your left hand) and lead her to pass on your right side. Step forward on 4 to gently check her movement with your left hand over your head, so that she will turn behind you to face your back.

Now lower you left hand on your left side. On 5-6-7&8, she will return to her starting position, doing a half turn to right, passing on your left side.

You will stay on the same spot facing forward throughout, pulsing and doing the regular Lindy footwork, although you can move a bit to left or right if necessary to give her more space as she circles around you.

The 6-count version of the Lasso is similar but faster.

Wrap-Around (8c)

The Wrap-Around is similar to the Lasso, but here you will lead the follower around you in a circle while keeping your left hand at waist level. Put your right hand on your heart as your left arm wraps around your waist. Keep the hand connection with the follower until 4 to let a stretch develop which will make her turn behind your back and return to her original position on your left side on 5-6-7&8. Catch her hand again at the end.

Stay on the same spot facing forward throughout, although you can move a bit to left or right if necessary to give her more space as she circles around you.

If you step diagonally back and to the right on 5, this will lead her into an outside free spin (right turn) on 5-6.

Quick Stop Drop (8c)

This popular move is a variation of the "Swingout with follower's outside turn on the back end", and also a great way to mark a break in the song or the end of a dance.

Do the first half of the Swingout (1-4). To lead the Quick Stop Drop, initiate the follower's outside turn earlier than usual, on 5, and then interrupt her turn and check her movement by quickly bringing your left hand down and bending your knees on 6-7. Freeze on 8.

She will complete her outside turn abruptly on 6-7, bend her knees and end up in a low, back-leaning position, facing you with her legs crossed, freezing on 8.

There is no triple-step on 7&8. The footwork on 4 to 8 is "step-step-step-hold".

This ending position requires a strong connection between the two of you which she can use as leverage. Lean back a little to give her a counter-weight.

Reverse Swingout (8c)

This is a fun variation on the regular Swingout. This time you will swing out the follower on your left side, not on your right side.

Start from a closed, side-by-side position, holding hands. Do a forward rock step (opposition break) while she does a regular rock-step, then on 3&4 lead her to triple in front of you and face you. The last step of your own triple (4) will be with your left foot diagonally back and behind your right foot, turning a quarter to left and clearing her way for the upcoming swingout. Stepping back will also give you a good stretch on her back with your right hand. Keep her close to you and make use of the momentum created by the forward rock step.

On 5-6, do a rock step (stepping back on right foot) while swinging out the follower to pass you on your left. Lead this with your right hand on her back. On the last triple-step turn left again to face the follower and end in an open position (7&8).

This step often surprises the follower which is good for breaking the monotony of too many predictable steps.

You can also try the Reverse Swingout from open position.

Around the World (8c)

This figure is similar to a Swingout with a free spin to right for both the leader and the follower.

Do a rock step in open, face-to-face position, with normal handhold. On the first triple step, approach each other turning slightly right, preparing to pass. Meanwhile, swing your right arm in a vertical circle, back low and forward high, and land your right hand (gently) on the follower's left shoulder on 4. With your left hand, lead her to continue into an underarm right turn as she passes you. As she turns, let go of her and make a full right spin yourself as well. After your mutual spins, reconnect face to face with normal handhold. You have now traded places.

This move looks like you are turning her with your right hand on her shoulder, but this is just an illusion. Let your right hand fall off her shoulder as she turns, without pulling.

Depending on your follower's ability, she can do a double free spin instead of a single one.

A common add-on to this figure is for both dancers to do the "Points" on the next 8 counts. As you spin and complete the Around the World, swing your right arm in a vertical circle again but in the opposite direction so that your hand swings up and forward on 1. Bend your right leg (back leg), maintain your weight on it, and point and wag your index finger at each other on 1-2, away on 3-4, and at each other again on 5-6-7-8.

Reverse Texas Tommy (8c)

Start in side-by-side closed position. Do a rock step. On 3&4, turn face-to-face and switch her right hand to your right hand behind her back. On 5, do a rock-step on RF and lead an inside underarm turn (right turn) with your right hand. Check her turn with your right hand on 6, and lead a hands-free outside turn (left turn) on 7&8.

You will lead this figure mostly with your right hand. She will turn twice in quick succession (to right and to left), while you are not turning at all.

Sailor Kicks (2 x 8c)

This fun figure will put you back-to-back with your partner, keeping a double handhold throughout.

It has two parts: first to get back-to-back, and then to walk in a circle doing kick-steps.

Start in face-to-face open position with double handhold. On the rock step (1-2), push your left hand forward and pull your right hand back to turn her slightly to her right. On the triple step (3&4), move towards her and swing both arms in the reverse direction (L back, R forward) to swing her back to her left and wind her up for a turn. On 5-6, take two small steps forward, turn a quarter to left and "roll her at your back" with a wide, sweeping motion of your left hand forward and over your head, landing on your left shoulder. The motion is similar to swinging a jacket at your back. Keep your right hand low and maintain the double handhold.

This will turn her back-to-back with you in a slightly offset position. She will be behind your right shoulder. You will hold her left hand with your right hand down at your right side, and her right hand with your left over your left shoulder. The handhold is loose, fingers resting on each other. On 7, finish this turning motion by dropping your knee slightly and freezing there for 8. She will do the same.

Be careful with this move (especially with a new partner) to avoid injury to shoulders or back. Keep your arms and your hand connection very relaxed and do not force anything.

On the next 8 beats, you will both walk around clockwise in a circle in this back-to-back position, using kick-steps, grove walk or other footwork. Unwind by letting go of your right hand, and turning 180 to left to face her in an open position.

The footwork is:
- Rock-step (1-2) / triple step (3&4) / step-step (5-6) / drop-hold (7-8)
- Kick-step-kick-step-kick-step-kick-step

Sugar Push (4c, 6c or 8c)

This common figure is danced face-to-face and can be done on 4, 6 or 8 counts. It consists of pulling in the follower face-to-face, compressing against her hand, then sending her back using the spring effect of the compression.

The 4-count version is quick and simple. Stand fairly close to each other. From an open position, lead a rock step (1-2). On 3, step forward on left foot and lead her to step forward as well. Offer your right hand (palm leading, fingers pointing to side), meet her left hand, and compress against it, checking the forward motion of both of you. Lean slightly into the compression. On 4, both of you bounce back to your original positions using the momentum of the compression. The footwork is "rock-step-step-step". The "push" happens on 3.

The 6-count version is the most common variant and it uses the familiar "1-2-3&4-5&6" pattern. Instead of a rock step, take two very small steps back and pull the follower into two forward steps (1-2). She can add swivels to her steps. The "push & check" action happens on 3&4: triple-step in place, offer your right hand and lean into the compression. On the second triple step, stay in place while she uses the momentum of the compression to travel back to her original spot (5&6).

To do an 8-count Sugar Push, send her back on 5-6 and do a triple-step or a Heel Pop on 7&8.

There are many variations of the Sugar Push. If you lift your left hand on 3, you can lead a tuck turn on "&4" (or on 5-6 in the case of the 8-count version). You can turn a quarter to left on 1-2 and press your right hand against her left hip on 3, replacing the hand compression. The Sugar Push can also be lead with double handhold.

Barrel Roll (6c)

Like many figures, the Barrel Roll can be done in 6-count or 8-count versions. It is a left side pass with mutual underarm turns, the follower doing a left underarm turn while the lead doing a right turn under his own arm, creating the illusion of the two bodies "rolling" against each other. For the same reason, the step is also referred to as "Car Wash".

Start the 6-count Barrel Roll from a face-to-face open position with normal handhold. Do a rock step (1-2). On 3&4, triple forward, first lower your left hand then make a half turn to right while raising your hand up over your head in a wide half-circle. This will lead the follower to do one and a half turns to her left while passing you on your left side. On 5&6, lower your hand and triple-step in place, face to face. You have now changed places.

The "roll" happens on 3&4 and it is a quick action. It is important that you start leading the turn in time by first lowering your hand. This will initiate her turn.

The Barrel Roll can also be done starting from a side-to-side closed position.

You can add one more turn for the follower on the second triple step (5&6). In this case, do not lower your hand when the first turn is over. Leave it up, lead the second turn, and lower your hand only at the end of the second triple step.

The Barrel Roll can also be led from an open position with a right-to-right "handshake" handhold. On the first triple step, lower and then raise your right hand up and across your chest and over your head. This will lead both of you to turn: she left, you right. Let her turn slightly ahead of you to avoid bumping your shoulders.

Barrel Roll (8c)

The 8-count Barrel Roll starts from an open position with a normal handhold.

It is very similar to the 6-count Barrel Roll from normal handhold but it is easier because there is more time available to complete the figure. Most of the turning will occur on 5-6 and you will have the last triple step (7&8) to comfortably finish the move.

Bow Tie (6c)

Also known as "Double Overhead Loop" or "Cross Arm Slide. Start in an open, face to face position, with double handhold.

Do a rock step (1-2). On 3&4, triple forward and lift both of your arms high. She will also triple forward and pass on your right side. Since your arms are up high, she will pass under your right arm and you will pass under your left arm.

On 7&8, you will both drop your hands behind your heads, release your handhold, and turn a quarter to right to face each other. Let your right hands slide down on each other's arm and catch her hand at the end, finishing with a right-to-right handhold.

This is also a good way to switch handholds in preparation for a move that requires cross handhold.

Double Tuck Turn (6c)

This is the same as the normal 6-count Tuck Turn, except on the second triple step you will lead two fast underarm turns (instead of one): the first on 5 and the second on 6.

For the follower, completing two full turns within one triple step is challenging, so try this step only if you know she can do it.

Hammerlock Turn (2 x 6c)

This figure consists of two 6-count parts.

The first part is a Tuck Turn starting from a face-to-face open position with double handhold.

Do a rock step (1-2). Raise your left hand on 3&4, and lead a tuck turn on 5&6 while maintaining double handhold. Keep your left hand up and hold her left hand with your right hand (reaching across between you and resting on her right side).

In the second part, you will untangle the hammerlock by leading a Change of Places with double handhold. After her turn on 3&4, you can maintain the double handhold or release your right hand to get into normal handhold. If you release your right hand, you can lead a second inside turn on 5&6.

Frankie's Sixies (3 x 6c)

This is a short chain of three 6-count figures (hence the name), often danced by Frankie Manning.

First 6-count: Start in open, face to face position with cross (R2R) handhold. Lead a Change of Places with underarm turn and do not let go of your right hand. On 5&6, cut in front of the follower in a tandem position (showing your back) and move to right so that she

99

moves to your left side behind your back. Take her left hand with your left hand while holding on to her right hand behind your back.

Second 6-count: Do a rock step together, and let go of your right hand (1-2). Now both of you triple forward on 3&4-5&6. As you move forward, both of you will do a gradual half-turn toward each other (you to left, she to right), ending up side-by-side again but facing the opposite direction. As you line up to her side, put your right hand around her waist.

Third 6-count: From here, lead a hands-free Tuck Turn, catch her hand and finish the figure in open, face-to-face position.

The Drag

Also referred to as "Tango Drag", implying that this is a borrowed step. Not to be confused with the blues dance called Slow Drag.

The Drag requires frontal body contact, chest-to-chest, body to body, so make sure that your follower is comfortable with this.

The Drag is essentially walking backwards in even steps (no triple-steps), with your stepping knee bent and weight kept on the back foot. You hold the follower in a close embrace and she walks with you, her knees also bent and weight on her forward foot, creating the impression that you are dragging her with you.

To get into this "Drag position", start from an open, face to face position with normal handhold (double handhold and R2R also work). On 1-2, do a forward rock step while swinging your left arm forward. This turns her slightly to her right and winds her up for a left turn. On 3-4, lead an inside (left) underarm turn and do a step-step in place (not a triple step). It is a step-step for her too.

On 5, catch her in a close embrace as she completes her turn, pick her up a little, and step back on left foot with flexed knee but leaving your right leg stretched out. Pull her to step forward on right foot, with knee bent. At the same time, push your left hand forward (holding her right hand). This is quite a lot to do in one beat, so it will take some practice to coordinate your limbs. Hold on 6.

From here you will walk backward, stepping on every second beat. First step back on right foot (1) maintaining the same pose but pulling back your left arm. Step back on left foot (3), swinging your left arm forward again. You can vary slows (stepping on every second beat) and quicks (stepping on every beat).

The Drag position looks like the follower is leaning on you, but in fact she should support her own weight on her forward foot. Her right arm should be completely relaxed to avoid discomfort as you swing it back and forth, much like in the Paddle.

To exit, step forward on right foot (5) and make a 180 turn to left to get into a side-by-side closed position with your follower (she is on your right side). Step back on 6, do a triple-step on 7&8, and you are ready for the next figure.

This particular sequence adds up to 14 beats, but the count is flexible and depends on the number and rhythm of the drag steps and the different ways of entering and exiting the figure.

The Drag is also a great way to end a dance, in which case you can just "drag" your partner off the dance floor.

Bonus Charleston figures

Tandem Charleston (8c-C3)

Also known as "Back Charleston". In this figure the leader lines up behind the follower and they perform the Lindy Charleston footwork pattern "in tandem", with double handhold.

Because of the geometry of the tandem position, the dancers must align their footwork (i.e. start on the same foot). To do this, one of the dancers has to switch their footwork when entering or exiting the tandem.

Getting into Tandem

There are many ways to get into Tandem Charleston.

You can easily get into Tandem position in just 4 beats, using the 4-count Tandem Turn. Start in an open position and do a rock step on 1-2. On 3, kick to side with left foot and pull the follower's right hand across in front of you in an arc, leading her into a half left-turn in front of you. On 4, hold your left foot in the air and pass her right hand into your right hand as she completes her half-turn, now backing you. If you started with a right-to-right handhold, then you will not need to pass her hand. Grab her left hand as well, and you are now in Tandem position.

Your footwork is "rock-step-kick-hold" and hers is "rock-step-step-hold", so that in this version she will be the one switching her footwork. At this point both of you will have your left foot free.

The second way to get into Tandem position is by doing an 8-count "Fake Tuck Turn". Start from side-to-side closed position. On 1-2, do a rock-step. On 3-4, prepare a tuck turn but don't raise your left hand (step-&). On 5-6, tap forward with your right foot and extend your left hand, winding her up for a left turn (tap-&). On 7-8, step to the side on right foot and pull her with your left hand into a half left turn and into Tandem position (step-&). Switch her hand into your right hand as she turns. Your complete footwork is: "rock-step-step-&-tap-&-step-&".

A third way to get into the Tandem Charleston is by doing a "Chase" (also called "S-Turn" or "Reverse Tuck Turn"). This is a longer, 10-count move (6c+4c). From closed position, do a 6-count Charleston Tuck Turn, except on the second kick-step (5-6) turn to right and face away, to the opposite direction.

Do another kick-step forward while she does a rock step backward, creating a stretch (7-8). Turn back towards her doing a last kick-step while she makes a half turn into Tandem position (9-10). Switch hands as she turns. Your complete footwork will be: "rock-step-kick-step-kick-step, kick-step-kick-step".

Doing the Tandem Charleston

Your footwork is the 1930s "Charleston for Lindy" footwork: "rock-step-kick-step-kick-&-kick-step".

Keep your hands low and palms-up, without gripping. She will place the palm of her hands on yours, without gripping. Both of you need to keep your arms and the handhold loose and relaxed to avoid strain or injury. Keep her hands at her side and don't pull them behind her back. Since she cannot see you, the hand connection is the only signal she receives from you.

Swing your arms naturally, left arm forward on 1 and 5, right arm forward on 3 and 7, just like in the Charleston Basic. You do this holding her hands.

Lean forward a little and keep your weight on the ball of your feet. Kick somewhat to the side to avoid kicking the follower. With some practice, you can dance the Tandem Charleston very close to each other without any accidents.

Try gradually rotating with her to left and to right to add variety to the basic Tandem Charleston.

Exiting the Tandem

There are several ways to exit the Tandem Charleston.

You can quickly exit in just 2 beats, on 5-6 of the Charleston Basic. On 5, as both dancers kick forward with their right foot, let go of her left hand and raise your right hand over her head prompting her to turn a quarter to her left. On 6, step down on right foot while she completes another quarter turn. You are now both ready for a rock step in open position with right-to-right handhold.

You can also exit by transitioning to Pancake Charleston. On 3, release your left hand, and swing your right hand in a big arc over her head counter-clockwise to lead an overhead turn to left. Bring your hand down quickly and let go of it, allowing her to do a 1¾ turn to left. You will do a 1¼ turn to left, using the momentum of your lead. Both of you will turn on left foot and keep kicking with right foot (usually 3 x kick-&) until you catch her right hand with your right hand in a Pancake position. From here continue with Pancake Charleston.

It is a natural transition from Tandem to Pancake because the leader and follower start on the same foot in both figures.

You can also exit using the follower's 180 turn, described further below.

Tandem Kick-Away (C3)

This is a repetitive step, similar to the Kick-Through Charleston or the Airplane Charleston, but done in a tandem position. Also called "Shadow Charleston". From a Tandem Charleston, you will both turn to right to kick away to right, and turn to left to kick away to left.

Get into Tandem Charleston. After a rock-step, immediately lead the kick-away to right by lifting your left hand and reaching over your follower's shoulder, turning both her and yourself a quarter to right. Maintain the double handhold. You are now side-by-side (she on your left) with your left hand over her shoulder, facing a quarter to right from your original direction. Kick forward on 3 and step down on LF on 4.

On the next 4 beats, both of you will turn 180 to left: kick forward with RF (5), pivot 180 to left on LF (6), kick forward with RF (7), and step down on RF (8). You are now side-by-side (she on your right) with your right hand over her shoulder, facing a quarter to left from your original direction.

 Repeat the kick-aways, left and right, a couple of times. The footwork will be a repeated "kick-turn-kick-step".

To transition back into Tandem Charleston, wait for a kick-away to right. After you step down on LF (4), stay facing that direction and do the next "kick-&-kick-step" in place while leading her to "kick-&-kick-step" in front of you, back into the Tandem position.

From here, do a rock step and you are back in Tandem Charleston. Note that you end up facing about a quarter to right compared to your original direction.

Tandem Push-Out (8c-C3)

Also called "Tandem Yo-Yo" as you will roll the follower out to face you and roll her back into Tandem, just like a yo-yo.

Release your left hand and put it on the follower's back during 1 of the rock step, and start pushing on 2 ("rock-push"). On 3-4 (kick-step) she will jump forward and turn 180 to right to face you. Maintain the right-to-right handhold with a stretch on 5 and bounce her back on 6 ("kick-pull") with a U-shape hand movement similar to the one used when entering the Tandem. She will jump forward again, turning 180 to left, back to Tandem position. Grab her left hand again on 8 and swing it forward on the rock step as usual.

There is no change to your usual Charleston Basic footwork throughout.

Follower's Half Turn (8c-C3)

This is the follower's half turn to left while doing the Tandem Charleston. It is often used to exit the Tandem.

While doing the Tandem Charleston, on 3 release your left hand and lift your right hand in a circle above her head, leading her into a left turn. Do not turn yourself. As soon as she completed the half turn (on 5), switch her hand from your right hand into your left hand, signalling that she should not turn further. You are now in a face-to-face open position.

Your footwork will be the normal Charleston Basic footwork, but hers will be "rock-step-kick-step-kick-&-kick-&", which allows her to switch legs so that she can start the next move on her right foot.

Follower's Full Turn (8c-C3)

This is the follower's full left turn in place, inserted into the Tandem Charleston.

Keep doing your regular Charleston Basic footwork throughout and do not turn.

Initiate her turn on 3 (the first kick) by lifting your right hand in a circle above her head. You have to let go of her left hand to allow her to turn, but catch it again as soon as she completed a full 360° turn, and lead her back into Tandem Charleston. She will have completed her turn by 7 (the final kick).

Charleston Boomerang (8c-C2 or C3)

This is the same as the Lindy Hop Boomerang, but done with either C2 or C3 Charleston footwork.

Charleston Swingout (8c-C2)

This is a Swingout starting from side-by-side closed position, replacing the triple steps with kick steps (C2). If the music is too fast, you can replace the kick-steps with groove steps.

Since the kick step (or groove step) generally covers less distance than a triple step, the Charleston Swingout will be tighter than a Lindy Swingout and less likely to cover a full 360 turn.

Flying Charleston (8c-C3)

This is a Charleston Swingout using the Lindy Charleston (C3) footwork. It can be danced either from a side-by-side closed position or from a face-to-face open position.

When starting from an open position, the "kick-step" on 3-4 is replaced by a "jump-step". This jump or hop forward on the supporting leg is used because a kick step covers less distance than a triple step, so it would be difficult to get close enough to the follower. Both of you will jump forward on 3, you on your right foot, she on her left. Use the stretch of the initial rock step to build momentum for the jump.

After the jump (3), both of you will step forward and pivot 180 to right, you on LF, she on RF (4). Swing her out on 5-6-7 while continuing to pivot 180 on your left leg (kick-&-kick). You will pivot on one spot and she will be hopping away from you to get back to her original position. Step back on RF on 8.

Note that there are several other steps out there that go by the name "Flying Charleston".

Double Charleston (2 x 6c-C4)

This figure is a combination of two 6-count Charleston Circles and adds up to yet another Charleston Swingout variation. You will dance this figure face-to-face throughout.

Do a 6-count Charleston Circle starting from open position. After the rock step (1-2), jump-step forward and pull her into closed position while making a quarter turn to the right (3-4). Continue turning another quarter in closed position on the second kick-step (5-6).

The rock step of the second 6-count Charleston Circle is done in closed position facing each other (1-2), giving each other a good stretch. On the subsequent two kick-steps continue turning to right and release her into open position.

Dancing the Lindy Hop

After learning and practicing the basics steps, the next challenge is to step up to the next level and become a competent social dancer.

Tempo of the music

When you start going out to dance socially, the first major issue you are likely to encounter is the tempo of the music you are trying to dance to.

At group Lindy classes, the music played is pleasantly mid-tempo. But when the beginner goes to his first social dance, he will be surprised to find that much of the music played comes in two varieties: too slow or too fast for him to dance the steps he learned in class. Even after taking more classes, the problem of tempos outside his comfort zone persists.

The heart of the problem is that not all music, including swing music, is suitable for dancing. Swing music can be danceable or not. This mainly depends on the tempo of the music, but also on other factors such as long introductions, erratic and unstable rhythms, long instrumental solos and other "irregularities".

Arguing about and judging swing music as danceable or not is nothing new. The Savoy dancers of the 1930s had constant discussions among themselves about the famous swing bands of the day and they each had the bands and songs they liked or disliked dancing to.

As a rule of thumb, the vast majority of music is not written with dancers in mind and the vast majority of the consumers of music are not dancers. Most composers and musicians are not dancers either, and they generally do not like to be confined by the needs of dancers. To a musician, predictable dance music is boring music, and in his mind a normal person would sit down and pay attention to the music, not jump around and create a distraction.

Every dance however, by its nature requires some predictability in the music, and a certain range of appropriate tempo (generally measured in beats per minute, or BPM). In that suitable range, the figures of the dance and the interaction between the dancers can be carried out in a deliberate and purposeful way. Outside that range, the dance will feel (and look) either comically rushed or grotesquely slow.

Ballroom dancing recognized this issue long time ago and resolved it with the concept of "strict tempo". Music played at ballroom classes, social dances and ballroom competitions must fall within a certain range of tempo and have some other prescribed characteristics. Strict tempo for Jive, for example, is 140-180 BMP. Strict tempo is a reasonable concept and it puts dancers first.

No such concept exists in Lindy Hop. Live bands in particular are prone to playing music that is either too fast or too slow for social dancing, but most DJ's are not much better and they seem to play anything as long as it has "swing" somewhere on the cover.

Since you generally cannot change the music at social dances, and assuming that you do not want to sit out 80% of the songs, you will then need to learn to cope with slow and fast music.

Pick the dance to the tempo

Every time the music starts, you have to make two quick decisions:

1) Do I want to dance to this piece of music?
   And if the answer is yes, then:
2) What type of dancing is suitable to the tempo of this music?

110

Swing dancing has many varieties and each variety is naturally suited to a certain tempo of music. Some of these swing dances (with the optimal range of beats per minute indicated in brackets) are, from slow to fast:

> Blues (40-80 BPM) → Foxtrot variants, Savoy style "Ballrooming", Slow Balboa (80-120 BPM) → Lindy Hop (120-160 BPM) → Lindy Hop with Charleston footwork, Jive, East Coast Swing (140-180 BPM) → Single-time Jive/ECS (160-200 BPM) → Classic Charleston, Breakaway, Balboa (180-220 BPM)

In this list, Foxtrot differs from the other dances because it is a progressive (travelling) dance while all the others are stationary (spot) dances. Foxtrot originates from the 1920s. It is a "trotting" ballroom dance of many variants, danced moving counter-clockwise on the dance floor, which is difficult to do when everyone else is dancing a spot dance. So Foxtrot is rarely an option at a Lindy Hop party.

There are still more swing dances like the Slow Foxtrot and Quickstep, which are not listed here because they are difficult ballroom dances not suitable for social dancing.

But even without these, there are plenty to choose from. Given the variety of swing dances, it should always be possible to find the right dance to a given tempo. The dances listed above cover most of the tempos played. And if the music gets excruciatingly fast or slow, one can always take a break and use it to rest and refresh.

Mid-tempo music

At a Lindy Hop social dance, if the swing is pleasantly mid-tempo, you will probably want to dance Lindy Hop.

Fast music

The practical response to faster music is to keep your steps smaller and tighter, your partner closer, your pulsing shallower, and to cut out any "unnecessary" body movements (like triple steps) where possible.

A common approach to dancing to faster swing music is: "just dance the Lindy Hop faster". This can result in some frenetic, exhausting and borderline comical dancing that may work for professional dancers or those under 20, but for everyone else, there is a more mature solution: pick a dance that suits the tempo of the music.

The swing dances that suit fast music best are the Classic Charleston, the Breakaway and the Balboa.

As the tempo increases, one may first switch from Lindy footwork to Lindy Charleston. It is easier to dance to faster music using Charleston footwork because it has no triple steps. The variety of the Charleston "kick-step" patterns can however present a challenge.

As the music gets even faster, you can try dancing in single steps, start incorporating Classic Charleston and Breakaway elements, and eventually switch to Balboa.

Balboa is probably the finest solution to the challenge of fast swing music. It is a fast, yet elegant, restrained and economical dance, danced in closed embrace in an upright position.

Slow music

Dancing to slow swing music is in some ways more difficult than fast dancing.

Fast dancing only requires a good sense of rhythm and good technical execution. But slow music leaves one more "exposed" because each figure takes a longer time to complete and the longer time frame needs to be filled with something. This requires greater balance and more precise control over your muscles. Whatever you do is more clearly visible.

The general approach to dancing to slower music includes increasing the smoothness and fluidity of the movements and completing each movement to the fullest, without holding back. The timing of the movements should be stretched out and a certain time delay should be introduced, where your steps happen just after the beat, and not right on the beat.

Slow dancing in swing draws from a few main sources: Lindy Hop danced slower, Slow Blues (or Slow Drag), Savoy style "Ballrooming", Slow Balboa, and Slow Jazz (or "fusion" dancing).

When the music gets slower, the Lindy Hopper's first reaction is to dance the same Lindy Hop figures, only slower. Stretch out the movements and add a certain time delay. Replace rock steps with forward steps. All this works to some extent, but at some point it starts to get awkward.

When the music gets really slow, some dancers switch to "slow blues dancing". Slow blues dancing originates from the Slow Drag that was danced "on a dime", in very tight close hold in the juke joints of the American South, and migrated to the big cities of the North at the beginning of the 20th century.

The Slow Drag mainly consists of shifting weight from one foot to the other with a time lag, perhaps in a step-tap format, and gyrating the hips with slightly bent knees in a tight close hold, earning the nickname "the grind". Modern-day proponents of blues dancing profess to do this with a sense of "deep respect of personal space" etc, which generally means that grinding is tamed into fake or pretend grinding. It is still not recommended to try this at your friendly neighbourhood Lindy Hop party.

Since the Slow Drag was not allowed at commercial dance venues, the dancers at the Savoy Ballroom faced the same question we do: What to dance to impossibly slow swing music? The answer they came up with was "Ballrooming". Ballrooming consists of assuming a loosely taken ballroom dance position, and shuffling around imitating some ballroom dance steps. To this day, this remains a viable (and fun) option.

You may also be able to find a local dance club that offers lessons in what is referred to as "slow jazz" or "fusion" dancing. As the name indicates, fusion dancing not an actual dance. It a mishmash of the Slow Drag, twisting, squirming and other assorted contortions, as well as steps borrowed from various dances and adapted to slower music. It is a means to facilitate "self-expression" without the trouble of learning a proper dance. It is danced mostly to monotonous, hard driving music in the 80 BMP range, to music without any perceptible beat, and seemingly to any music that was never intended to be danced to. Try it and see if it gives you any ideas to deal with slow music.

Just like Balboa on the fast end, Slow Balboa is probably the best dance to try on the slower spectrum of swing music. Slow Balboa originated at the same place and around the same time as Balboa, but it is not a slower version of it. It is a different, graceful dance that itself has a number of styles or variants.

Variety and playfulness

There are various ways of keeping Lindy Hop from becoming boring and going stale, including:

- Using a good mix of figures of varying beat count and complexity

114

- Choosing steps that vary the type and direction of body movement (circular vs linear, turning right vs left etc.)
- Applying footwork variations
- Giving space to your partner to express herself and do her favourite jazz steps
- Doing your own jazz steps and variations
- Surprising your partner, for example with interrupted and redirected steps

Ideally, all this should be done in harmony with the music and applied where the music calls for it.

Lindy Hop is often perceived as a rotational dance, mostly because of the emphasis placed on the Swingout as the signature move of the dance. But in reality, the Lindy is a dance of "circles and lines", and a balance should be kept between the two.

Endless turns and rotations, especially in the same direction, will quickly become boring for everyone and can cause dizziness. Breaks and separations for jazz steps are a welcome change. Figures that have a different direction or speed of movement, like the He-Goes-She-Goes, Cat Walk, Sailor Kicks, Jig Kicks, Reverse Swingout, Washing Machine or Switches can also break the monotony. The tempo of the music will of course set some limits to the techniques you can use.

It is important to pay attention to the ending of each figure. Usually there is a choice for setting up a subsequent rotation versus a subsequent linear move, and you need to prepare for this ahead of time. An example could be the Lindy Circle. If you finish it with a triple-step backwards, a linear move will follow more naturally. If you finish it still rotating, a rotational move will fit more naturally.

Musicality

Once you get involved with Lindy Hop, you will soon start hearing about "musicality" or "musical interpretation". This primarily refers to the structure of a song, and the ways a dancer may shape his dancing to conform or respond to the structure of the music.

As a swing dancer, it is useful to have some familiarity with the typical structure and the basic building blocks of swing music. The reason for this is that dance is a physical expression of the music, the music drives the dance and, ideally, one "dances to the music". To dance to the music, one needs to understand the music at least to some degree. This does not mean that you have to be a musician or know musical theory but having a certain awareness of the structure of a song helps in "molding" your dance to it.

Having said that, "musicality" is sometimes over-emphasized in Lindy instruction at the expense of teaching and drilling steps. As a beginner Lindy Hopper, you probably don't need to be overly concerned with musicality for two reasons. First, it is difficult to focus on this kind of thing when you are still not sure where to put your feet in the first place. Second, the majority of your dance partners will not know what "musicality" even is, and if they do know they probably do not care too much about it.

In the beginning, therefore, the focus should be on learning the basic steps well and on keeping the rhythm of the music. If you can do this, you are already a dancer. When dancing starts to become second nature, that is the time to work on the finer points of musicality.

In the quest for dancing the Lindy Hop with musicality, variety and playfulness, the ultimate is "improvisation".

Improvisation

The essence of jazz music and jazz dancing is improvisation. The problem is, it is not easy to tell what improvisation is in the first place, and so this chapter will be more like brainstorming than clear explanation.

A good starting point could be the dictionary which defines improvisation as "the act of making or doing something with whatever is available at the time." In dancing, "whatever is available" generally includes your body, the music, the steps you know, your dance partner, and the dance floor. Using these tools, one can experiment with shape, time, speed and energy in forming a dance.

Leading a good variety of steps, applying footwork variations, and adding break steps is all good dancing, but it is still not improvisation. A dance planned out ahead of time is not improvisation. In order to improvise, one needs to step out of the confines of learned figures and make the dance their own. Repeating certain learned patterns is just a recital; improvisation starts where one can through himself into the music to "see what happens".

Dancing steps that one was not planning to do, in response to the follower, to the music, or to the conditions on the dance floor, creating spontaneously steps that the follower can still follow are elements of improvised dancing.

Other than the necessity of reacting to unforeseen events, the main driving force behind improvisation is the effort to fight off boredom. As complicated as a dance appears to be to the beginner, once it is mastered it becomes increasingly simple to do, and therefore increasingly boring to do. To break the boredom, one has to come up with something new, something unexpected, something ingenious.

Improvisation is also defined as using intuition in applying some learned skills. So for a dancer to be able to improvise, he still has to have solid technical skills and needs to know well a number of the identifiable steps of the dance.

Improvisation could mean taking apart figures, breaking them down to their smallest (generally 2-beat) components, and putting the parts back together differently, so that it still makes sense. For example, one can look at a basic 8-count figure as two empty boxes consisting of the same pattern: step-step-triple-step. What can these boxes be filled with, based on what you already know about Lindy Hop so that it adds up to something new and meaningful?

Repetitive steps are good tools to use in improvisation, and the simplest "repetitive dance" is the One-Step. It is worthwhile so study it and use it to add some silly fun to your dancing. The One-Step takes us back to the early 20th century when new dances were invented almost by the month. Dances were not considered sacred rituals of prescribed steps. Anyone could and did come up with a new dance. So why not assume a mindset of trying to come up with a new dance to the music played at the next Lindy Hop party.

To improvise a dance, one will of course need a good follower who is able to react to the lead spontaneously, using her own intuition. A good follower will often have the need to improvise on her own, and when both dancers try to improvise at the same time, that's when the real fun begins.

Ending a dance

Ending a dance when the music stops is easy enough as you can simply "stop dancing". However, there are ways to make the ending feel more fun and look much better. Here are a few suggestions:

- End the song with a Quick Stop Drop.

- Use a Side Slide, for example on the second half of a Lindy Circle, to break the momentum and slow down the dance for the ending.
- Use the Drag to "drag" your partner off the dance floor.
- Separate for break steps towards the end of the song and use the final 4 beats to do a Lock Step with a spin and hold.

If you want to use an explicit ending move, it is important to correctly match it to the end of the song as it can look silly if you do it too early or too late relative to the music.

Practice routines

It is a common challenge for the beginner leader to try and put together figures so that they form a coherent dance for the duration of a song. This challenge is not unique to Lindy Hop and the leader faces the same issue in any non-choreographed social dance.

Until you develop a certain level of mastery where you have figures stored in muscle memory and no longer have to consciously think of the steps you dance, it can be useful to have a few "fall-back" routines or step combinations memorized. This is a crutch, and it is better not to use them for very long, but it sure beats going blank in the middle of a dance.

A few random routines are shown below. Use them if they are any helpful to you, or make up your own based on the steps you already know or want to learn. Each line of these routines fits the common 8-bar (32-beat) musical "phrase" of swing music. 6-count figures are shown in italics.

Because these are practice routines, they have a high concentration of steps. When dancing socially, do not use them on your follower all at once. Pick a line or a particular sequence, memorize it and add it to your social dancing, blended with basic steps. Planned dance routines, or pieces of it, are also good for practice with a partner.

Medium tempo music

1. Lindy Circle, Swingout, Swingout with inside turn, Lindy Circle
2. *Tuck Turn (6c), Belt Turn (6c), American Turn (6c), Right Side Pass (6c)*, Swingout
3. Lindy Circle with Side-Chassés, Change of Places (8c), Cuddle (8c), Heel Taps (8c)
4. Lindy Circle, Double Tuck Turn, Frisbee to side-by-side (8c), Lindy Circle

5. Lindy Circle, *Tuck Turn (6c), 2 x Sugar Push (6c), Change of Places (6c)*
6. Swingout with Jump Stop, Lowdown (8c), Lindy Circle, She-Goes
7. *Tuck Turn (6c), 6-count Frisbee (to R2R handhold), Overhead Loop (6c), Change of Places (6c)*, Applejacks (8c)
8. Swingout, Boomerang, Swingback, Lindy Circle

9. Tuck Turn Push-Around, Swingout, Swingout with outside turn on exit, Lindy Circe
10. Swingout with Texas Tommy, *Right Side Pass (6c), Frankie's Sixies (3x6c)*
11. *Change of Places (6c), Chicken Walk (6c), Sugar Push (6c), Change of Places (6c)*, Boogie Drops (8c)
12. Lindy Circle, Promenade, Swingout, Lindy Circe with front-end inside turn

13. Swingout, Lasso, Swingback, Lindy Circle
14. *Rollout (6c), Sugar Push (6c)*, Lindy Circle, *Hammerlock Turn (2x6c)*

15. *Cuddle (2x6c), Bow Tie (6c), Right Side Pass (6c)*, Lindy Circle
16. Swingout (overturned), Switches (8c), Swingout, Tacky Annie (8c)

17. Around the World with Points (2x8c), Lindy Circle, Reverse Swingout
18. *Hands-free Tuck Turn (6c), Barrel Roll (6c), Washing Machine (14c), Right Side Pass (6c)*
19. Jazz Box (2x8c), Trucking (8c), Fishtail (8c)
20. Fakeout, Swing-Not, Swingout, Swingout with Quick Stop Drop

Faster music

1. 2 x Charleston Basic, Skip-Up, Peel-Away to side-by-side (4c), Freeze (4c)
2. Charleston Basic, 2 x Charleston She Goes, Charleston Circle,
3. *2 x Jig Kicks (6c), Charleston Tuck Turn (6c)*, Charleston Cuddle (8c)
4. 2 x Flying Charleston, Charleston Circle, Charleston Basic

5. Charleston Basic to Kick-Through, Kick-Through, Kick-Through Free Turns to Left & to Right
6. 3 x Hand-to-Hand Charleston, Butterfly
7. *Charleston Tuck Turn (6c), Double Charleston (2x6c), Charleston Side Pass (6c)*, Charleston Swingout
8. Charleston Circle (C3), 2 x Charleston Swingout, Charleston Circle

9. 2 x Charleston She-Goes, 2 x Charleston Basic
10. 2 x Airplane Charleston, 2 x Hand-to-Hand Charleston
11. 2 x Kick-Through, 2 x Airplane Charleston
12. Skip Up (8c), Peel Away to open position (8c), Sailor Kicks (2x8c)

Leaders and followers

One of the benefits of social dancing is that one gets to know many new people and gets to dance with a variety of followers.

For a successful partner dancing experience, the leader must lead fairly well and the follower must follow fairly well. But since followers come with different talents, abilities, experience levels and attitudes, you generally won't be able to predict what to expect from a follower who you have never danced with before.

Here are some general observations about leaders and followers.

Experience levels

Followers at a social dance come at all levels of experience, and often you will not be able to judge the experience level of a new dance partner until you start dancing with her. For this and other reasons, it is better to start each dance slow and easy and only gradually increase the complexity of the steps.

It will be soon evident whether your follower is a beginner, or she is approximately at your level, or she is a better dancer than you are.

If she is a beginner, it is best to dance at her level, to lead simple steps and to let her practice what she appears to already know. This may not be very satisfying for you, but there is no point in forcing something that will probably not work. Instead, focus on the social aspect of dancing with a new person. However, if she can clearly keep the rhythm and follow your lead easily, you may try some more complex steps.

Dancing with someone at your level (for example a current or former classmate), is generally both satisfying and useful. It will not have the constraints of dancing with a total beginner, nor the stress of dancing with an advanced dancer.

If your partner is the better dancer, then you are as much at her mercy as the beginner is at your mercy. Just as you can confuse the beginner by leading steps she cannot follow, the experienced follower can confuse you with doing footwork variations or extended step variations that you did not expect. If she is kind, she will follow your lead and dance to your level. This is a good experience to have, dancing with someone who easily follows what you are trying to lead. If she is not so kind, or if it shows that she'd be rather dancing with a better dancer, then just focus on your lead and ignore what she does.

The good follower

When dancing with a partner, your own dancing will necessarily be affected by the movement, weight, strength, timing and momentum of another body. If your partner dances well, everything falls into place in harmony, momentum transfers smoothly without the need for force, and your movements are mutually supported by each other. If she does not dance well, than you will have to find a way to successfully deal with another body that is trying to frustrate what you do.

Generally this is what a leader is hoping for when dancing with a stranger:

- A good follower will wait for and focus on the lead and not guess or anticipate what step is coming next. This enables the follower to react instantaneously and to follow figures she has never danced before.

Many followers have difficulty with this concept and it is not entirely their fault as in class, leads and follows are typically taught the same way: 'This is the figure and this is how you should do it'. But leaders and followers do not dance the same way. Leaders initiate a figure and they foresee the step which will follow, before it happens. Followers see none of this. They dance based on quick, immediate external signals and don't even know how the current figure will end let alone the next. This basic difference in dancing is often not made clear to the followers, and so they learn to guess what is coming next based on the steps they know. If they guess incorrectly, the dance will fail. Even if they guess correctly, often the follow will get ahead of the lead and the dance is not a communication; it is two people talking at the same time.

If there is no signal from the leader, a good follower will either do nothing (other than pulsing) or if she is currently engaged in a movement she will continue that movement. For example, if she is doing a turn she will continue repeating that turn in the absence of a lead to stop it.

This does not mean that a follower has no freedom during the dance. She does have plenty as discussed in the next section.

- An extension of the previous point is that the good follower will not be fazed by any unexpected moves. She will react curiously and switch to an appropriate movement of her own.

- The follower should generally keep her own balance, including during turns and spins, not lean on the lead and not expect the lead to support her weight. She has an easy touch so that dancing does not turn into wrestling.

- The partners will often use stretch or compression to leverage on each other. The good follower is ready to give you a solid frame when it is called for. It is difficult to lead a follower with "spaghetti arms".

- The movement of the good follower is smooth and flexible. She may be energetic and decisive but not rigid or jerky.

- The good follower will give you a relaxed hand connection with any tension only in the fingers. This allows for smooth adjustment of hand positions and hand contact during turns or separations. It is difficult to separate or change handholds when the follower grips your hand.

- When the good follower is led into a free turn, she will keep her hands at approximately the same level and position where you let go of them, so that you can easily catch them at the end of the turn. In most cases this will be at waist level. On your part, you should also keep your hand at about the same position where it was when you released contact.

Leading a good follower is like driving a sports car: quick, nimble, agile, breaks well, responds to every input immediately and precisely. Dancing with a poor follower is more like driving a bus.

<u>Freedom of the follower</u>

While the leader generally leads the dance and chooses the figures, the follower has considerable freedom in Lindy Hop. She can use this freedom in several ways.

She can of course apply her own styling and footwork variations. This should not impact the lead at all.

The follower can "break away" from the lead, for example at the end of a Swingout, and dance some jazz steps on her own. Either the leader or the follower can then offer to connect again.

Finally, the follower can interrupt a lead and perform a turn or step on her own initiative. This means temporarily taking over the lead. This turns the dance into a real dialogue or give-and-take, but it is also certain to confuse an inexperienced lead.

It depends on the follower how much of this freedom she wants to use. Many will never use the freedom they have and are happy to just follow. If you give them too much space, they will feel left alone and think that you are not doing your job. Other, usually experienced, followers will use this freedom a lot.

It follows then that the leader should not be preoccupied only with leading steps. He should always watch for the interpretation of the dance by the follower and give her the space that he thinks she requires. An experienced follower is not only led by you – she is also led by the music.

The good leader

As dancers, we obviously want to be good leaders but the ultimate judges of who a good leader is are the followers we dance with.

If you ask followers what they consider to be the characteristics of a good leader, they will usually say that a good leader is the one who wants to give the follower a good dance experience. A common complaint from followers is that many leaders dance as if the follower is not even there.

Therefore, Rule No. 1 for the leader is: care about your follower and don't just dance for yourself.

The following are some more specific points on being a good leader:

- The good leader pulsates expressly (not so shallowly that the follower cannot feel it) and keeps the rhythm of the music correctly.
- The good leader initiates every lead clearly and at the right time, without ambiguity or hesitation.
- The lead is fluid, the follower never feels that the flow of the movement stops (unless the stop is deliberate).
- The good leader gives space to the follower to do her own variations and break steps, but not so much that she feels she is dancing alone.
- The good leader pays attention to what the follower is doing, responds to her playfully and has an ongoing "dance conversation" with her.
- Followers appreciate the occasional new and fancy step if it is not overdone.

Followers seem to appreciate different strengths in the various leaders they dance with. In other words, every good leader is good for some unique reason.

Other than clear and unambiguous lead, each follower seems to have their own expectations and preferences, which means that there is not one "perfect way" to lead. No matter how good one is, he will not be a perfect lead for everyone. And if you do not dance regularly with a follower, you will not be able to guess what she likes.

The bottom line is that you should have good technique, clear lead and early "calibration" with your dance partner, including her experience level and how she responds to certain moves. If it works out well, great. If not, you did all you could, so just move on to the next follower.

The picture and the frame

Partner dancing has always had an unwritten rule. It may sound old school but one will rarely go wrong by following it. It has been said that a dancing couple is like a painting: the man is the frame and the lady is the picture. Whether you like it or not, anyone looking at a dancing couple will mainly look at the lady.

So as a leader you have a decision to make before you even start to dance: If your objective is to shine with fancy steps and cool styling, chances are that you will be soon marked as a show-off. If your objective is to make your partner look good and feel good, it is virtually guaranteed that you will be a sought-after dancer.

Social dancing

Going to a swing dance is usually a light-hearted experience. The music is lively and happy and people are generally friendly. With that said, your satisfaction level will likely vary from evening to evening depending on various factors which you either can or cannot control. Some dances and some evenings will just turn out better than others.

Also, going to a dance for the first time can be intimidating. You will see leaders at various experience levels and it may appear that everyone there is a much better dancer than you are. This is generally not the case and there is no need to be overly impressed with the seemingly fancy steps you see. You will soon start to realize that they are just common steps you are simply not yet familiar with.

Type of the social dance

Since swing dances come in many varieties, a social swing dance will tend toward one or the other based on the organizers' preferences. A typical social swing dance will focus on either Lindy Hop or East Coast Swing/Jive. For a Lindy Hopper, the first type is of course ideal. East Coast Swing events tend to play more of 1950s rock and roll / rockabilly music and they are a good opportunity to practice 6-count steps and learn some new ones. West Coast Swing, however is a significantly different dance, hardly a swing dance despite the name, and the West Coast Swing scene tends to be separate from the Lindy Hop scene.

Recurring dances are organized by dance schools, swing dance or music associations, entertainment venues or community centres. It is easy to obtain information on these events and on upcoming classes and workshops on the organizers' websites and on social media.

It is often announced in advance who the DJ will be, or whether a live band will be playing. This is useful information as you will soon develop a feel for which DJ and band tends to play the kind of music you prefer.

<u>The crowd</u>

At any given social dance there will be many people present, and you can dance with any follower. In theory.

The people present will generally fall into one of a number of informal groups. There will be the experienced dancers or teachers who know each other and may gather in one area. These are the regulars and some of them may just come to chat with each other and catch up on the latest. They may not dance much, and if they do they may prefer to dance among themselves.

There will be groups of friends who dance together, talk and laugh together and generally are into each other. They may not decline an invitation to dance but will spend the song waiting for the chance to get back to their friends.

Then there will be those who just heard about the event somewhere and came to check it out and attend the "free beginner class", or came to accompany someone. They don't actually know how to dance. They will not decline if you ask them to dance, but they may consider it your job to tell them what to do.

So while in theory you can dance with anyone, by the time you are done mapping out those who don't really know what they are doing, and the mini parties where you are not invited, you may find the number of your potential dance partners significantly reduced.

In general, the best dance partner is a follower who can dance at a certain level and comes alone with the express purpose of actually dancing – a less common specimen than one would hope. If you find them, get their names and seek them out in the future.

Finally, be aware that these days any expectation of privacy has all but disappeared and annoying phones or cameras staring into your face on the dance floor have become a standard nuisance. Chances are that the day after the dance you will find your pictures posted somewhere on the Internet, whether you like it or not.

Conditions on the dance floor

It is primarily the leader's job to keep an eye on the surroundings and protect his follower from accidents. You will need to adjust your dancing according to how crowded the dance floor is.

Walk your partner to a less crowded part of the floor and start the dance there in the first place. As you dance, the crowd will shift, so keep guiding your partner into the available space that opens up. Watch out for other dancers and keep away from those who dance recklessly or use large body movements. Ideally, your partner should also look out for you and warn you of any danger behind you by pressing your hand or pulling you a little, but you cannot rely on her doing this.

The more crowded the floor the smaller you need to keep your "dancing footprint". Limit backward movements and especially limit your kicks.

As you navigate the floor, make sure to stay away from the loudspeakers. Noise of just 90 decibels can permanently damage your hearing within two hours of exposure.

Teaching on the dance floor

Teaching on the dance floor comes in two varieties and neither is overly productive. Version 1 is when you try to teach your partner, and version 2 is when your dance partner is trying to teach you.

It is sometimes tempting to give unsolicited advice to your dance partner either because she is lost or because she dances poorly. I would recommend that you don't. At its core, correcting someone is a form of criticism and few people like to be criticised. Besides, you can never be sure that when something is not working it is the follower's fault and not yours. So just cover for her mistakes and make the most of the experience.

Sometimes a follower will ask you to teach her. It is best to politely decline. Just say that you are still learning this yourself. Teaching on the dance floor is a messy and pointless business with the loud music and all the people dancing around you, and you probably don't know how to dance the follower's part in any case. If she wants a lesson she can always take a class.

Receiving unsolicited advice from others, or asking others to teach you, are similarly ineffective.

However, you can learn a lot by simply observing others, taking note of what you like, trying to break it down and practicing it on your own. It is also a good idea to ask people where they learned certain things, and then follow up on that trail.

Stealing a dance and jam sessions

It is customary at some point during a social dance to form a circle and dedicate a dance to out-of-town participants or those who celebrate their birthdays. These celebrants will be called to the centre of the circle and the other dancers will take turns dancing with them for a short period of time (about 10-15 seconds) before passing them on to the next dancer. Those not dancing will be watching and clapping.

To jump in and "steal" the celebrant from the dancer who happens to dance with them is not difficult but a few tips can help make it smoother.

Prepare yourself by getting into the rhythm and starting to pulse, then step forward, into the circle to signal that you are "ready to steal". There could be others to step forward at the same time, so you will have to work out who is next. This happens naturally.

As a leader, you will steal a follower from another lead who is currently dancing with her, so get in sync with the lead and try to "shadow" him.

As far as timing is concerned, the best "entry point" is the end of an 8- or 6-count figure (i.e. beat 8 or 6). If you can get hold of the celebrant on that last beat, you are ready to continue the dance naturally with a new figure.

The key to a smooth entry is positioning. It is difficult, or impossible, to do a smooth takeover if you stand too far from the couple at the critical time, or too close, or behind the leader. Generally, it is easier to jump in from the couple's "open side" which is not blocked by their hands.

At the critical point you want to be either on the lead's right side or the follower's left side. Also, it is easier to loiter in one area and wait until the couple lines up, rather than running around and trying to get into a good position.

You can get hold of the follower in two ways: in open position (face-to-face) or in closed position (side-by-side). Watch the couple and anticipate where the follower will be next. Your goal is to be either face-to-face with the follower or have her on your right side at the point of takeover. If you steal in open position, take her hand in a normal left to right handhold. If you steal side-by-side, put your right arm around her waist. Take her gently but firmly so that she can feel the new lead.

Dance with the celebrant for 10-15 seconds and be mindful that certain figures (for example Lindy Circles) makes it more difficult for the next dancer to step in and steal. When you have passed the celebrant on to the next dancer, back away, join the circle and start clapping.

A jam session is similar to a birthday dance in that the dancers form a circle and let willing participants get in the middle and take turns showing off their talents for a short period of time (about 15-20 seconds). Couples can show their moves or individuals can show off their jazz steps.

Band nights

Supporting local jazz bands is a good cause, but "band nights" at social dances can be a mixed bag. While DJ's are generally mindful of the fact that people are trying to dance to their music (no guarantees), live bands tend to play only two kinds of music: too fast or too slow. They are often amateur musicians who are happy to have an opportunity to play to an audience, and usually play without much concern for the needs of the dancers.

Back in the old days, royal courts and commercial ballrooms could hire orchestras and professional house bands and tell them exactly what kind of music they should pay. But small local bands have a repertoire that they developed usually not with dancers in mind. They have to consider the musicians in the band, their availability and skill level, and to choose songs so that every member has something interesting to play, not necessarily music preferred by dancers.

If a swing dance event is a "band night", it is advisable to do some research about the band, or see them once for testing. If you find that at your current level you can't dance to most of what they play, either resign to the fact that you will be sitting a lot listening to good music, or skip that event and wait for a DJ'd dance. It will be cheaper and the tempo will probably be more suitable for your dancing.

The Shim Sham

This book is about partner dancing and it is not concerned with choreographed dancing. However, one exception can be made for the "Shim Sham" because it has become customary at social dances for all dancers to perform this routine during a break.

The Shim Sham is a short choreographed dance routine that has a number of variations one of which is shown below. It includes some steps not discussed in this book.

Traditionally, many jazz moves start on the last ("lead-in") beat (beat 8) of the preceding musical phrase, not on beat 1 like most regular steps do. In the Shim Sham routine, Tacky Annie and Boogie Forward start on 1, all other figures start on 8.

> *Shim Sham [6 bars], Full Break [2 bars]*
> *Push and Cross Over [8b]*
> *Tacky Annie [6b], Full Break [2b]*
> *Half Break [2b], Full Break [2b], Half Break [2b], Full Break [2b]*
>
> *Shim Sham [6b], Freeze [2b]*
> *Push and Cross Over [8b]*
> *Tacky Annie [6 bars], Freeze [2b]*
> *Half Break [2b], Freeze [2b], Half Break [2b], Freeze [2b]*

135

Boogie Back [2b], Boogie Fwd [2b], Boogie Back [2b], Boogie Fwd [2b]
Boogie Back [2b], Shorty George [2b], Boogie Back [2b], Shorty George [2b]
➔ *Grab someone near you and start dancing*

Other popular choreographed routines include the Tranky Doo, Big Apple, Jitterbug Stroll, Mama's Stew and Trickeration.

www.ingramcontent.com/pod-product-compliance
Lightning Source LLC
Chambersburg PA
CBHW071211020426
42333CB00015B/1373